Fun & Fitness For The Fine And Foxy and The Old School Players

(An Easy Guide to Staying Fit as We Age)

By

Bruce H. Dobbs

Advanced Certified Fitness Trainer

Elegantly written, here's a very necessary sermon about the author's lifetime journey in pursuit of physical fitness and overall well-being. This is a striking narrative that juxtaposes the author's personal origin story with his development as a nationally recognized physical fitness expert.... Adopting an existential and a wholistic approach towards the relationship between a healthy mind and a healthy body, the author has successfully crafted an extraordinary treatise on the fundamental importance of physical fitness as the perfect antidote to the stress and strain of 21st Century life. Go buy this book today." Donald E. Smart, Esq. Managing Partner THE SMART LAW FIRM Milford, Connecticut

Forward

We constantly speak about the health benefits of a well-planned timely orchestration of life's primary principles. We also frequently interject the finer inner wisdom that manifests itself within the totality of one's specifics. These concepts reveal themselves by carefully examining and activating them within the limitless boundaries of time, age, and intention. I am blessed to be the author's friend, teacher, and close cosmic brother. Let me say his theoretical and practical approach has been well demonstrated. Through thick and thin and hard work the one that stands above all else is that he has never lost sight of his unwavering commitment to being the best husband and father. All shows in the unshakable commitment and immense desire to help and share his knowledge wisdom and understanding with people from all walks of life and all parts of the world.

Pendekar, Bahati Mersant

Introduction

I am currently vice president of a biotechnology company that specializes in the development of drugs (nano antibodies to be specific) designed to treat and cure several diseases. I am also a certified advanced fitness trainer at one of the largest publicly traded fitness health gyms in the United States. My Biotechnology company's programs include oncology, immunology virology and ophthalmology. In my capacity I am privileged to be on the phone and in video conference calls with some of the most renowned scientists in their respective fields All of the scientists agree, and I know as a fitness trainer, that exercise diet and proper rest go a long way to, fighting inflammation, (a condition endemic to many diseases), and living a long and healthy life.

In the next few pages, I'll share with you what I've learned from some of the top internationally known scientists and what I've learned from my own research and experience. I am not a doctor, nor do I have a PhD in molecular biology nor am I attempting in any way shape or form dispensing medical advice. Before embarking on any exercise program or taking any of the vitamins or supplements described in this book, I urge you to consult your licensed physician or medical practitioner.

In fact, I am challenging you to become a student of your own health, a student of your own body. Each one of us is different and in my opinion part of being fit and being healthy involves knowing what works for you. This also entails taking care of your mental health.

Stress, anxiety, and depression are elements that can cause a breakdown of the physical body. While physical exercise can help with stress and anxiety, fighting depression may require the help of a professional as it is sometimes a herculean effort to climb out of the hole of negative thinking and depression.

My first impression of becoming aware of physical fitness came from as a child watching Jack Lalanne and Tarzan on television. In junior high school I used to love the part in gym class where we had to climb ropes. I had no idea that all the time I was building upper body strength. I am sure that the upper body strength I built during that time helped me to play African drums for hours and hours nonstop. In high school I studied Shotokan Karate with Houlon Willis, but it wasn't until my second year in college studying under Dr. Moses Powell and his system named Sanuces Ryu that I gained an appreciation for being fit. My other martial arts teachers are Vern Riddings, Francis Fong, Gary Mitchell, Taji Nanji, Cecil Siao-Pao, Billy White, Michael Reid, Phillip Ghee and Bahati Mersant. Interestingly my teachers became my personal friends and in the case of the last ten twelve years I learned high level intricacies and secrets hanging out informally in their living rooms, backyards, and garages. I learned the stuff not taught in formal class setting. Each taught me their individual styles and shared with me the lineage and history of their styles.

Kun Tao Silat, the martial art that was introduced to me by Phil Ghee and Bahati Mersant is what resonates most with me. Of all the styles that I have studied Kun Tao is like graduate school. All my martial arts teachers have told me to "take this and make it your own". It wasn't until I came into my own that I began to flourish in the art. So, I say to you take the information I share with you regarding fitness, health and wellness and make it your own.

For ongoing Information got to:
www.yourphenomenallife.net

Every Day Is A Holiday/Holy Day Every Meal Is A Feast!

Health And Wellness, The Decision to Act

If You Haven't Already, Here's How To Get On Your Own Path To Health And Wellness

It's not to late for you to get on your path to health and wellness. You can lose weight, gain muscle, lower your blood pressure, get your blood sugar under control, become more flexible, strengthen your bones, have more energy, and feel better mentally and physically. If you think you are too old or believe you are overweight because you are "Big Boned" (There is no such thing as being big boned. It a euphemism) or believe you don't have time, or you are to tired to exercise or whatever, perhaps now is the time to make another decision. There will always be an excuse.

The truth" s, research has consistently shown healthy Individuals, people with chronic conditions like diabetes and heart disease and even cancer patients can benefit from consistent exercise and a wellness lifestyle. The truth is you already know this stuff and nothing anyone says to you is going to launch you on your path or keep you on your path until and unless you make the decision.

Amelia Earhart said "The most difficult thing is the decision to act, the rest is merely tenacity. The fears are paper tigers. You can do anything you decide to do. You can act to change and control your life; and the procedure, the process is its own reward".

Howard Thurman wrote "It's a wondrous thing, that a decision to act releases energy in the personality. For days on end a person may drift along without much energy. Having no particular sense of direction and having no will change. Then, something happens to alter the pattern. It may be something very simple and inconsequential. But it stabs awake, it alarms, it disturbs. In a flash, one gets a vivid picture of oneself, and it passes. The result is a decision. Sharp, definitive decision. In the wake of the decision, yes, even as a part of the decision itself, energy is released. The act of decision sweeps all before it, and the life of the individual maybe changed forever."

Now that you have made the decision to act, know that a health and wellness lifestyle does not happen all at once. Know that lifestyle change happens gradually. It stars by tweaking the little things. You must discover what works best for you. For example, if you are an avid potato chip eater, you may look to replace the potato chips with a *healthy* vegetable chip. Continue to visit this site and you will find tips and tweaks to help you. You still will have to do some reading and experimenting to see what works for you.

> **Tip:** *Terra makes a good veggie chip that tastes good with guacamole. You can get those individual little guacamole cups so you don't waste an entire avocado.*

You don't need a gym membership, exercise equipment or designer exercise clothing to get started. All you need to begin is your body. As you continue exercise you will naturally want to acquire an exercise mat, a few dumbbells and maybe a jump rope. You can start with a fifteen-minute full-body work out with no equipment. Here is a fifteen-minute no equipment full body workout for beginners. You should consult with your doctor before beginning exercise or taking any kind of nutritional supplement.

Set a day to get started. Promise yourself that you will do at least fifteen minutes. Tell a friend or family member to act as a coach and hold your feet to the fire. For best results, if you have little grandchildren tell them you want them to coach you and ask them call you every day to make sure you exercised. Tell them you will pay them as a coach.

The Science of Fitness and Longevity

Fitness and longevity are two interconnected aspects of human health that have fascinated scientists and researchers for decades. The pursuit of a healthy and active lifestyle not only improves physical well-being but also enhances the prospects of living a longer, disease-free life. This chapter delves into the science behind fitness and longevity, exploring the physiological and molecular mechanisms that contribute to these desired outcomes.

1. **Physical Fitness and Longevity:** Physical fitness refers to the body's ability to carry out daily activities with vigor, without undue fatigue, and with ample energy reserves for emergencies. Engaging in

regular exercise and maintaining a healthy level of fitness has been strongly linked to increased longevity. Various studies have highlighted the following mechanisms through which physical fitness influences longevity:

a. **Cardiovascular Health:** Regular exercise improves cardiovascular fitness by strengthening the heart, improving blood circulation, and reducing the risk of heart disease. Physical activity helps maintain healthy blood pressure, lowers cholesterol levels, and reduces the likelihood of developing chronic conditions such as stroke, coronary artery disease, and heart failure.

b. **Metabolic Benefits:** Physical fitness positively impacts metabolism, contributing to weight management and reducing the risk of metabolic disorders such as diabetes. Regular exercise enhances insulin sensitivity, facilitates glucose utilization, and promotes a healthy balance of lipids in the body.

c. **Immune System Function:** Exercise has been shown to have immunomodulatory effects, bolstering the immune system's ability to fight infections and reducing the risk of chronic inflammation. This leads to a lower susceptibility to various diseases, contributing to overall longevity.

d. **Maintenance of Bone Health:** Weight-bearing exercises and resistance training play a crucial role in maintaining bone health and preventing age-related bone loss. By improving bone density and strength, physical fitness reduces the risk of osteoporosis and fractures, thereby enhancing longevity.

2. **Molecular Mechanisms of Longevity:** Beyond the visible benefits of physical fitness, scientists have delved into the molecular mechanisms that underlie longevity. Research in this field has identified several pathways and factors that influence the aging process and overall lifespan:

    a. **Telomeres and Cellular Aging:** Telomeres, protective structures at the ends of chromosomes, shorten with each cell division, leading to cellular aging. Regular exercise and a healthy lifestyle have been associated with longer telomeres, suggesting that physical fitness may slow down cellular aging and extend lifespan.

    b. **Caloric Restriction and Metabolic Pathways:** Caloric restriction, without malnutrition, has been shown to extend lifespan in various organisms. This dietary intervention triggers metabolic pathways such as insulin/IGF-1 signaling and the mTOR pathway, which regulate cellular processes related to aging and longevity.

c. **Oxidative Stress and Inflammation:** Oxidative stress and chronic inflammation are key factors in aging and age-related diseases. Regular exercise has been found to reduce oxidative stress and promote an anti-inflammatory environment, contributing to healthy aging and increased longevity.

d. **Hormesis and Adaptive Response:** The concept of hormesis suggests that exposure to mild stressors, such as exercise, can stimulate an adaptive response in the body, leading to improved resilience and longevity. This response involves the activation of cellular repair mechanisms, antioxidant defenses, and stress resistance pathways.

The science of fitness and longevity continues to evolve, uncovering intricate connections between physical activity, molecular mechanisms, and lifespan. Engaging in regular exercise and maintaining physical fitness offers numerous benefits, including improved cardiovascular health, metabolic balance, immune system function, and bone health. Furthermore, understanding the molecular pathways associated with longevity provides valuable insights into how lifestyle factors, such as exercise, can impact the aging process. By incorporating fitness into our daily lives, we can enhance our overall well-being and strive for a longer, healthier, and more fulfilling life.

Energy production in cells involves several molecular pathways. The primary pathway responsible for generating energy is called cellular respiration, which occurs in the mitochondria of eukaryotic cells. Cellular respiration involves three main stages: glycolysis, the Krebs cycle (also known as the citric acid cycle or TCA cycle), and oxidative phosphorylation.

1. **Glycolysis:** This is the initial step in energy production and occurs in the cytoplasm. It involves the breakdown of glucose, a six-carbon sugar molecule, into two molecules of pyruvate, a three-carbon compound. Glycolysis yields a small amount of ATP (adenosine triphosphate) directly and also generates NADH (nicotinamide adenine dinucleotide) as a high-energy electron carrier.

2. **Pyruvate Decarboxylation:** After glycolysis, pyruvate molecules produced are transported into the mitochondria. In the mitochondrial matrix, each pyruvate molecule is converted into acetyl-CoA (acetyl coenzyme A) in a process called pyruvate decarboxylation. This step generates more NADH.

3. **Krebs Cycle:** Acetyl-CoA enters the Krebs cycle, which takes place in the mitochondrial matrix. In this cycle, acetyl-CoA is oxidized, releasing high-energy electrons and producing ATP, NADH, and FADH2 (flavin adenine dinucleotide). The high-energy electrons are carried by NADH and FADH2 to the next stage.

4. **Oxidative Phosphorylation:** The final stage occurs in the inner mitochondrial membrane. It involves the transfer of electrons from NADH and FADH2 to a series of protein complexes called the electron transport chain (ETC). As the electrons pass through the ETC, their energy is used to pump protons (H+) from the mitochondrial matrix to the intermembrane space, creating an electrochemical gradient. The energy stored in this gradient is then utilized by ATP synthase, an enzyme complex, to produce ATP through a process called chemiosmosis. This is known as oxidative phosphorylation because ATP synthesis is coupled with the transfer of electrons (oxidation) and the phosphorylation of ADP (adenosine diphosphate) to ATP.

In summary, glucose is broken down through glycolysis and pyruvate decarboxylation, generating NADH. Acetyl-CoA is then produced and enters the Krebs cycle, yielding NADH, FADH2, and a small amount of ATP. The high-energy electrons carried by NADH and FADH2 are transferred to the electron transport chain, leading to the generation of ATP through oxidative phosphorylation.

It's Important to note that other molecules, such as fatty acids and certain amino acids, can also enter these energy-producing pathways at different stages, contributing to the overall energy production in cells.

Aging is an inevitable process that affects all living organisms, including human beings. As we grow older, our bodies undergo numerous changes at the cellular, tissue, and organ levels. This three-page essay aims to explore the various aspects of aging, including the underlying mechanisms, the effects on different body systems, and the potential interventions to mitigate its impact. Understanding aging is crucial for developing strategies to promote healthy aging and improve the quality of life for individuals as they grow older.

I. **The Biology of Aging**: Aging is a complex biological process influenced by both genetic and environmental factors. At the cellular level, aging is characterized by several key mechanisms, such as telomere shortening, mitochondrial dysfunction, and the accumulation of cellular damage. Telomeres, the protective caps at the ends of chromosomes, gradually shorten with each cell division, ultimately leading to cellular senescence. Mitochondria, the powerhouses of the cell responsible for energy production, undergo functional decline with age, leading to decreased energy production and increased oxidative stress.

II. **Effects on Body Systems:**

   a. **Musculoskeletal System:** One of the noticeable effects of aging on the musculoskeletal system is a loss of muscle mass and strength, known as sarcopenia. This contributes to decreased mobility, increased risk of falls, and frailty in older individuals. Additionally, aging bones become more fragile, leading to a higher susceptibility to fractures and osteoporosis.

b. **Cardiovascular System:** The cardiovascular system undergoes age-related changes that can result in various conditions, including hypertension, atherosclerosis, and heart failure. Blood vessels lose their elasticity, leading to decreased blood flow and increased blood pressure. The heart muscle becomes stiffer and less efficient, reducing its ability to pump blood effectively.

c. **Nervous System:** Aging affects the nervous system, leading to a decline in cognitive function and an increased risk of neurodegenerative diseases such as Alzheimer's and Parkinson's. The brain undergoes structural and functional changes, including reduced volume and impaired neurotransmitter signaling. These changes can result in memory loss, decreased cognitive flexibility, and slower information processing.

d. **Immune System:** The immune system undergoes age-related changes known as immunosenescence, leading to a decline in immune function. This can result in increased susceptibility to infections, reduced response to vaccinations, and an increased risk of autoimmune diseases and cancer.

III. **Interventions for Healthy Aging:** While aging is a natural process, there are interventions that can help promote healthy aging and reduce age-related health issues. These interventions include:

    a. **Regular Physical Activity:** Engaging in regular exercise, including aerobic activities and strength training, has been shown to improve muscle strength, cardiovascular health, and cognitive function. Exercise also helps maintain a healthy body weight, reduces the risk of chronic diseases, and improves overall well-being.

    b. **Balanced Diet:** Eating a nutritious diet rich in fruits, vegetables, whole grains, lean proteins, and healthy fats provides the necessary nutrients and antioxidants to support optimal health. Adequate hydration is also important for maintaining bodily functions.

    c. **Stress Management:** Chronic stress can accelerate the aging process and increase the risk of various health problems. Effective stress management techniques such as mindfulness, meditation, and relaxation exercises can help reduce stress levels and promote emotional well-being.

d. **Regular Health Check-ups:** Regular medical check-ups allow for early detection and management of age-related conditions. It is important to monitor blood pressure, cholesterol levels, blood sugar, and other health markers regularly to address any emerging issues promptly.

Understanding aging and its effects on the body is crucial for developing strategies to promote healthy aging and improve the quality of life for older individuals. By focusing on lifestyle factors such as regular physical activity, a balanced diet, stress management, and regular health check-ups, individuals can take proactive steps to mitigate the impact of aging and maintain their overall well-being as they grow older. Additionally, ongoing research in the field of aging biology holds promise for the development of novel interventions that may further enhance healthy aging in the future.

What is the role of inflammation in disease?

Inflammation plays a complex and important role in the development and progression of various diseases. While inflammation is a natural response of the immune system to protect the body from harmful stimuli, such as infections and tissue damage, chronic or excessive inflammation can contribute to the pathogenesis of many diseases. Here are some key points regarding the role of inflammation in disease:

1. **Acute Inflammation:** Acute inflammation is a short-term response that aims to eliminate the initial cause of injury, remove damaged cells, and initiate tissue repair. It involves the release of chemical signals, dilation of blood vessels, and recruitment of immune cells to the affected area. Acute inflammation is usually beneficial and necessary for healing.

2. **Chronic Inflammation:** When inflammation persists over a long period or becomes dysregulated, it can lead to chronic inflammation. Chronic inflammation is associated with various diseases, including autoimmune disorders (e.g., rheumatoid arthritis, inflammatory bowel disease), cardiovascular diseases (e.g., atherosclerosis), neurodegenerative diseases (e.g., Alzheimer's disease), metabolic disorders (e.g., obesity, diabetes), and certain types of cancer.

3. **Immune Dysregulation:** Inflammatory responses involve a complex interplay between immune cells, signaling molecules (cytokines), and various mediators. In some diseases, the immune system becomes dysregulated, leading to an exaggerated or inappropriate immune response. This can result in tissue damage, organ dysfunction, and the perpetuation of inflammation.

4. **Tissue Damage:** Prolonged inflammation can lead to tissue damage and fibrosis. Inflammatory cells, such as macrophages, can release enzymes and reactive oxygen species that harm surrounding tissues.

Additionally, chronic inflammation can disrupt normal tissue repair processes, leading to the accumulation of scar tissue and impaired organ function.

5. **Disease Progression:** Inflammation can contribute to the progression of certain diseases. For example, chronic inflammation in atherosclerosis leads to the formation of plaques and narrowing of blood vessels. Inflammatory processes in cancer can promote tumor growth, invasion, and metastasis. Inflammatory responses in autoimmune diseases can result in the destruction of healthy tissues.

6. **Therapeutic Target:** Recognizing the role of inflammation in disease has led to the development of therapies targeting inflammation. Anti-inflammatory drugs, such as nonsteroidal anti-inflammatory drugs (NSAIDs) and corticosteroids, are commonly used to alleviate symptoms and reduce inflammation in various conditions. Additionally, biologic therapies that specifically target inflammatory molecules or immune cells have been developed for specific diseases.

It is important to note that while inflammation is often associated with disease, it is also a crucial part of the body's defense mechanism against infections and injuries. Proper regulation and resolution of inflammation are necessary for maintaining overall health.

What Happens Chemically within our bodies when we exercise?

When we exercise, several chemical processes occur within our bodies to support the increased demand for energy and to maintain homeostasis. Here's a simplified explanation of the main chemical reactions and processes that take place during exercise:

1. **Energy production:** The primary source of energy during exercise is adenosine triphosphate (ATP). ATP is generated through different metabolic pathways depending on the intensity and duration of exercise:

    a. **Aerobic metabolism:** During low to moderate-intensity exercises, such as jogging or brisk walking, the body relies on aerobic metabolism. This process occurs in the mitochondria of cells and involves the breakdown of carbohydrates (glucose) and fats (fatty acids) in the presence of oxygen to produce ATP. The chemical reactions involved are glycolysis, the Krebs cycle (also known as the citric acid cycle or TCA cycle), and oxidative phosphorylation.

    b. **Anaerobic metabolism:** During high-intensity exercises, like sprinting or weightlifting, the body switches to anaerobic metabolism. In this case, ATP is generated without the presence of oxygen through a process called glycolysis. Glycolysis breaks down glucose into pyruvate and produces a small amount of ATP. If oxygen availability is limited, pyruvate is converted into lactate, resulting in the accumulation of lactic acid. This buildup of lactic acid contributes to muscle fatigue.

2. **Oxygen consumption:** As exercise intensity increases, the body's demand for oxygen rises. Oxygen is transported to exercising muscles through the bloodstream by binding to hemoglobin in red blood cells. In the muscles, oxygen is utilized by mitochondria to support aerobic metabolism and the production of ATP.

3. **Respiratory and cardiovascular response:** During exercise, the respiratory and cardiovascular systems work together to deliver oxygen to the muscles and remove waste products. The respiratory rate and depth increase, enhancing the intake of oxygen and the elimination of carbon dioxide. Simultaneously, the heart rate and stroke volume increase, leading to an elevated cardiac output. These responses ensure sufficient oxygen supply to the working muscles and help remove metabolic byproducts.

4. **Hormonal regulation:** Exercise triggers the release of various hormones that regulate energy metabolism, blood glucose levels, and other physiological processes. For example:

a. Epinephrine and norepinephrine (adrenaline and noradrenaline) are released from the adrenal glands, promoting the breakdown of glycogen (stored glucose) in the liver and muscles, as well as increasing heart rate and blood flow.

b. Insulin levels may decrease during exercise, allowing more glucose to be available for energy production.

c. Growth hormone (GH) and testosterone levels may increase, stimulating protein synthesis and muscle growth.

5. **Heat regulation:** During exercise, the body generates heat as a byproduct of energy production. To maintain normal body temperature, mechanisms such as sweating, and vasodilation (widening of blood vessels) occur. Sweating helps dissipate heat through evaporation, while vasodilation enhances blood flow to the skin, facilitating heat loss.

It's important to note that these processes are interconnected and influenced by factors like exercise intensity, duration, and individual fitness levels. This explanation provides a general overview of the chemical changes that occur in the body during exercise but does not cover all the intricacies and details involved in physiological responses.

To assess your current fitness level, you can follow these steps:

1. **Define your fitness goals:** Determine what you want to achieve with your fitness routine. Are you aiming to improve cardiovascular endurance, strength, flexibility, or overall fitness? Having clear goals will help you measure your progress accurately.

2. **Assess cardiovascular endurance:** Cardiovascular endurance measures how efficiently your heart and lungs deliver oxygen to your muscles during prolonged exercise. You can evaluate it by performing activities such as running, swimming, cycling, or using a cardio machine (treadmill, elliptical, etc.). Monitor your heart rate, time, and intensity during these activities to gauge your endurance level.

3. **Evaluate strength:** Strength assessment involves measuring the force your muscles can exert. You can perform exercises like push-ups, squats, lunges, or weightlifting to evaluate your strength. Keep track of the number of repetitions or the amount of weight you can lift for different exercises.

4. **Test flexibility:** Flexibility refers to the range of motion in your joints and muscles. To assess flexibility, try various stretches that target major muscle groups, such as hamstring stretches, shoulder stretches, or yoga poses. Note any limitations or discomfort you experience during these movements.

5. **Measure body composition:** Body composition indicates the proportion of muscle, fat, bone, and other tissues in your body. While it doesn't directly measure fitness, it can provide insights into your overall health. Methods for assessing body composition include measuring body mass index (BMI), skinfold calipers, bioelectrical impedance analysis (BIA), or dual-energy X-ray absorptiometry (DXA) scans.

6. **Consider other fitness indicators:** Apart from the above measurements, you can also assess other factors that indicate your fitness level. These may include balance, coordination, agility, and reaction time. You can evaluate these through specific exercises or tests related to each factor.

7. **Monitor your progress:** Regularly track your fitness activities and measurements over time. This allows you to see improvements, identify areas that need more focus, and adjust your fitness routine accordingly.

Remember, fitness is a multifaceted concept, and no single test can fully capture your overall fitness level. It's beneficial to consult with a fitness professional or personal trainer who can guide you through a comprehensive assessment and provide personalized recommendations based on your goals and abilities.

How long does it take to improve cardiovascular health?

The time it takes to improve cardiovascular health can vary depending on several factors, including your current fitness level, genetic predispositions, lifestyle choices, and the specific type and intensity of exercise you engage in. However, with consistent effort and a well-rounded approach, you can typically begin to see improvements in cardiovascular health within a few weeks to a few months. Here are some general guidelines to consider:

1. **Exercise Frequency:** Engage in cardiovascular exercise at least three to five times per week. Aim for a minimum of 150 minutes of moderate-intensity exercise or 75 minutes of vigorous-intensity exercise each week.

2. **Exercise Intensity:** Incorporate both moderate-intensity and high-intensity exercises into your routine. Moderate-intensity exercises include brisk walking, cycling, swimming, or dancing, while high-intensity exercises may include running, interval training, or vigorous sports.

3. **Duration:** Gradually increase the duration of your workouts over time. Begin with shorter sessions and gradually work your way up to 30 minutes or more per session.

4. **Variety:** Include a mix of aerobic exercises (e.g., jogging, cycling) and anaerobic exercises (e.g., weightlifting, interval training) in your routine. This

variety can help improve different aspects of cardiovascular fitness.

5. **Progression:** As your fitness improves, challenge yourself by increasing the intensity, duration, or frequency of your workouts. This progressive overload helps stimulate further cardiovascular adaptations.

6. **Healthy Lifestyle:** Support your cardiovascular health by maintaining a balanced diet, managing stress, getting adequate sleep, and avoiding tobacco use or excessive alcohol consumption.

7. **Consult a Professional:** If you have any pre-existing health conditions or concerns, it's important to consult with a healthcare professional or a certified fitness trainer who can provide personalized guidance and recommendations.

Remember that everyone's journey is unique, and individual results may vary. It's essential to listen to your body, start at a level that is appropriate for you, and gradually progress over time. Consistency and commitment to a healthy lifestyle are key to improving cardiovascular health.

How to strengthen the lungs through breathing exercises

To strengthen the lungs through breathing exercises, you can incorporate the following techniques into your routine:

1. **Diaphragmatic breathing:** Also known as deep belly breathing, this technique helps strengthen the diaphragm and increases lung capacity. Follow these steps:

   - Sit or lie down in a comfortable position.
   - Place one hand on your chest and the other on your abdomen.
   - Inhale deeply through your nose, allowing your abdomen to rise as you fill your lungs with air.
   - Exhale slowly through your mouth, letting your abdomen fall as you release the air.
   - Repeat for several minutes, gradually extending the duration of each inhalation and exhalation.

2. **Pursed lip breathing:** This technique can help improve the efficiency of breathing and decrease shortness of breath. Here's how to do it:

   - Sit or stand in a relaxed position.
   - Inhale deeply through your nose for a count of two.

- Pucker your lips as if you were going to blow out candles and exhale slowly and evenly through your mouth for a count of four.
- Repeat for several minutes, gradually increasing the duration of your exhalation.

3. **Breath-holding exercises:** These exercises can help increase lung capacity and train your lungs to utilize oxygen more effectively. Start with shorter breath holds and gradually increase the duration as you become more comfortable. Here's a simple exercise to try:

   - Inhale deeply through your nose.
   - Hold your breath for a count of 5 to 10 seconds.
   - Exhale slowly through your mouth.
   - Repeat several times, gradually increasing the duration of the breath hold.

4. **Interval training:** This involves alternating between periods of high-intensity and low-intensity breathing. It can help strengthen the respiratory muscles and improve overall lung function. For example:

   - Inhale deeply and rapidly for a short burst of intense breathing.
   - Exhale slowly and fully, allowing your breath to return to normal.
   - Repeat the cycle for a set duration or number of repetitions.

5. **Cardiovascular exercises:** Engaging in aerobic activities, such as brisk walking, jogging, swimming, or cycling, can improve lung capacity and overall respiratory fitness. These exercises challenge the lungs and heart, leading to stronger respiratory muscles and increased lung efficiency.

Remember, if you have any existing medical conditions or concerns, it's always best to consult with a healthcare professional before starting any new exercise regimen, including breathing exercises.

How long does it take to get stronger?

The time it takes to get stronger varies greatly depending on various factors, including your current fitness level, genetics, training program, nutrition, rest and recovery, and consistency. There is no one-size-fits-all answer, as everyone progresses at their own pace.

In general, noticeable strength gains can be observed within a few weeks to a few months of consistent and structured training. During this time, your body adapts to the demands placed on it, leading to increased muscle strength and neural adaptations.

However, significant strength improvements usually take several months to years of dedicated training, depending on your goals. It's important to remember that strength development is a gradual process that requires patience and perseverance.

To optimize your progress, consider the following tips:

1. **Consistency:** Regularly engage in strength training exercises, ideally at least two to three times per week. Make it a habit and stick to your training plan.

2. **Progressive Overload**: Gradually increase the demands placed on your muscles over time. This can be achieved by progressively increasing the weight, repetitions, or intensity of your workouts.

3. **Proper Technique:** Focus on maintaining proper form and technique during exercises to target the intended muscles effectively and minimize the risk of injury.

4. **Balanced Nutrition**: Ensure you're consuming a balanced diet that provides adequate protein, carbohydrates, and healthy fats to support muscle growth and recovery.

5. **Sufficient Rest and Recovery**: Allow your body time to recover between workouts. Get enough sleep, as it plays a crucial role in muscle repair and growth.

6. **Patience:** Building strength is a long-term endeavor. Embrace the journey and avoid comparing yourself to others. Celebrate small victories along the way and stay motivated.

Remember, it's always a good idea to consult with a qualified fitness professional or trainer who can design a personalized training program tailored to your goals and abilities.

How long does it take to become more flexible?

The time it takes to become more flexible can vary greatly depending on several factors, including your current level of flexibility, your age, genetics, and the amount of time and effort you dedicate to stretching and flexibility exercises. It is important to note that flexibility is a gradual process and requires consistent practice over an extended period.

With regular stretching and flexibility exercises, you can expect to see some improvement in your flexibility within a few weeks or months. However, significant gains in flexibility usually take more time and effort. It's important to approach flexibility training with patience and persistence.

To enhance your flexibility, consider incorporating the following practices into your routine:

1. **Stretching exercises:** Engage in regular stretching exercises that target the specific areas you want to improve. Static stretching, dynamic stretching, and proprioceptive neuromuscular facilitation (PNF) techniques are commonly used.

2. **Consistency:** Dedicate time each day or several times a week to stretch and work on your flexibility. Consistency is key to seeing progress over time.

3. **Gradual progression:** Start with gentle stretches and gradually increase the intensity and duration of your stretching sessions as your flexibility improves. Push

yourself within a comfortable range, but avoid overstretching or causing pain.

4. **Variety:** Incorporate a variety of stretching exercises and techniques to target different muscle groups and improve overall flexibility. This will help prevent plateaus and keep your routine interesting.

5. **Warm-up:** Prior to stretching, warm up your muscles with light aerobic exercise or by performing dynamic movements. This helps increase blood flow and prepares your muscles for stretching.

Remember that everyone's body is unique, and the rate of improvement in flexibility varies from person to person. Be patient, consistent, and listen to your body's limits to avoid injuries. If you have any concerns or pre-existing conditions, consult with a healthcare professional or a qualified trainer before starting a new flexibility program.

What is delayed onset muscle soreness?

Delayed onset muscle soreness (DOMS) refers to the muscular discomfort and pain that occurs after engaging in strenuous exercise or physical activity. It typically develops between 24 and 72 hours following the activity and is characterized by a dull, aching pain in the affected muscles.

DOMS is believed to be caused by microscopic damage to muscle fibers and the surrounding connective tissues. When you engage in intense physical activity, particularly exercises that involve eccentric muscle contractions (lengthening of the muscle under tension), such as downhill running or weightlifting, it can result in small tears in the muscle fibers. These micro-tears trigger an inflammatory response, leading to the symptoms associated with DOMS.

The exact mechanisms behind DOMS are not fully understood, but several factors are thought to contribute to its development, including:

1. **Muscle fiber damage:** Eccentric contractions, which occur when the muscle is lengthening under tension, are believed to cause more muscle fiber damage than other types of contractions.

2. **Inflammation:** The muscle damage triggers an inflammatory response in the body, involving the release of various chemicals and immune cells that contribute to the pain and discomfort.

3. **Metabolic waste accumulation:** During intense exercise, metabolic byproducts, such as lactic acid, can accumulate in the muscles. These byproducts may contribute to the soreness experienced later.

Symptoms of DOMS typically include muscle stiffness, tenderness to touch, reduced range of motion, and muscle weakness. The severity of DOMS can vary depending on factors such as the intensity and duration of the exercise, an individual's fitness level, and their susceptibility to muscle damage.

It's important to note that while DOMS can be uncomfortable, it is generally a normal response to intense exercise and is not typically a cause for concern. The discomfort usually resolves within a few days as the muscles repair themselves and adapt to the physical stress. To alleviate the symptoms, rest, gentle stretching, applying ice or heat, and taking over-the-counter pain relievers may provide relief. Gradually easing into new exercise programs and incorporating proper warm-up and cool-down routines can also help prevent or minimize the severity of DOMS.

How important is sleep when it comes to fitness?

Sleep is extremely important when it comes to fitness. It plays a crucial role in supporting overall health and well-being, including your physical performance, recovery, and muscle growth. Here are several reasons why sleep is essential for fitness:

1. **Muscle recovery:** During sleep, your body undergoes important processes such as protein synthesis, tissue repair, and the release of growth hormone. These processes are vital for muscle recovery and growth after exercise. Without sufficient sleep, your muscles may not have enough time to repair and rebuild, leading to decreased performance and increased risk of injury.

2. **Energy levels and performance:** Sleep deprivation can significantly impact your energy levels and athletic performance. Lack of sleep can impair cognitive function, reaction time, coordination, and decision-making skills. These effects can hinder your ability to perform at your best during workouts or sports activities.

3. **Hormonal balance:** Sleep plays a crucial role in regulating hormone levels that affect fitness and body composition. Insufficient sleep can disrupt the balance of hormones like cortisol, which is associated with stress, muscle breakdown, and fat gain. Additionally, inadequate sleep can lower levels of growth hormone and testosterone, both of which are important for muscle growth and recovery.

4. **Appetite regulation and weight management:** Lack of sleep can disrupt the hormones that control hunger and satiety, such as leptin and ghrelin. When these hormones are imbalanced, it can lead to increased appetite, cravings for unhealthy foods, and a higher risk of overeating. Poor sleep has also been linked to weight gain and an increased likelihood of obesity.

5. **Injury prevention:** Sleep deprivation can impair your coordination, balance, and reaction time, increasing the risk of accidents and injuries during physical activities or workouts. Adequate sleep helps ensure that your mind and body are alert, reducing the chances of accidents and helping you perform exercises with proper form and technique.

To optimize your fitness goals, it is recommended to prioritize sleep and aim for 7-9 hours of quality sleep per night. Establishing a consistent sleep schedule, creating a sleep-friendly environment, and adopting good sleep hygiene practices can all contribute to better sleep and improved fitness outcomes.

What is the science behind weight loss?

Weight loss is a complex process that involves various physiological and biochemical factors. The science behind weight loss revolves around creating an energy deficit, where the energy expended exceeds the energy consumed. This deficit prompts the body to utilize stored energy, primarily in the form of body fat, resulting in weight loss. Here are some key factors involved:

1. **Energy Balance:** Weight loss ultimately depends on the balance between energy intake (calories consumed through food and beverages) and energy expenditure (calories burned through basal metabolic rate, physical activity, and other bodily processes). To lose weight, you need to create a calorie deficit by either consuming fewer calories or increasing physical activity, or a combination of both.

2. **Basal Metabolic Rate (BMR):** BMR refers to the number of calories your body requires to maintain basic functions at rest, such as breathing, circulation, and cell production. BMR accounts for a significant portion of daily energy expenditure. Factors that affect BMR include age, sex, body composition, and genetics.

3. **Diet:** A balanced, nutritious diet plays a crucial role in weight loss. Reducing calorie intake by consuming a calorie-deficient diet can lead to weight loss. It is generally recommended to focus on whole, unprocessed foods, including fruits, vegetables, lean proteins, whole grains, and healthy fats.

Additionally, portion control and mindful eating practices can help manage calorie intake.

4. **Physical Activity:** Increasing physical activity helps burn calories, contributes to weight loss, and improves overall health. Engaging in both aerobic exercises (e.g., running, swimming) and strength training (e.g., weightlifting) can be beneficial. Exercise not only burns calories during the activity but can also increase metabolic rate and preserve muscle mass, which aids in weight management.

5. **Hormonal Factors:** Hormones like insulin, ghrelin, leptin, and cortisol influence appetite, metabolism, and fat storage. For example, insulin regulates blood sugar levels and promotes fat storage, while ghrelin stimulates hunger. Understanding how these hormones work can help in developing effective weight loss strategies.

6. **Genetics:** Genetics can influence individual variations in metabolism, fat storage, and appetite regulation. Some individuals may have a genetic predisposition to store excess fat or have a slower metabolism. However, genetics do not determine one's destiny, and lifestyle modifications can still lead to successful weight loss.

It's important to note that sustainable weight loss is a gradual process, and crash diets or extreme measures are generally not recommended. Consulting with a healthcare professional or a registered dietitian can provide personalized guidance based on your specific needs and goals.

How many calories must you burn to lose one pound?

To lose one pound of body weight, you generally need to create a calorie deficit of approximately 3,500 calories. This means that you would need to burn 3,500 calories more than you consume. However, it's important to note that weight loss is influenced by various factors such as individual metabolism, body composition, and overall health.

It's generally recommended to approach weight loss in a gradual and sustainable manner. Aiming for a moderate calorie deficit of 500 to 1,000 calories per day is often considered safe and effective. By creating this daily deficit, you can expect to lose about 1-2 pounds per week.

Keep in mind that weight loss is not solely determined by calories burned through exercise. Your overall energy balance, which includes both calorie intake and expenditure throughout the day, plays a significant role. A combination of a healthy, balanced diet and regular physical activity is typically recommended for safe and sustainable weight loss. It's always a good idea to consult with a healthcare professional or a registered dietitian before starting any weight loss program to receive personalized advice.

How much water should you drink every day?

The amount of water a person needs to drink each day can vary depending on various factors such as age, sex, activity level, and overall health. The general recommendation for daily water intake is often referred to as the "8x8 rule," which suggests drinking eight 8-ounce glasses of water, equal to about 2 liters or half a gallon. However, this is a rough guideline and may not be suitable for everyone.

In recent years, there has been a shift towards a more individualized approach to hydration. The National Academies of Sciences, Engineering, and Medicine in the United States provides general recommendations, stating that men should aim for about 3.7 liters (about 13 cups) of total water intake per day, while women should aim for about 2.7 liters (about 9 cups) of total water intake per day. This includes fluids from all sources, including beverages and food.

It's important to note that these recommendations include all fluids, not just water. Additionally, certain circumstances may increase the need for more water, such as hot weather, intense physical activity, or certain health conditions. It's always a good idea to listen to your body's signals of thirst and adjust your water intake accordingly.

Remember that individual needs can vary, so it's best to consult with a healthcare professional who can provide personalized advice based on your specific circumstances.

What is the difference between a macronutrient and a micronutrient?

Macronutrients and micronutrients are two categories of essential nutrients required by the human body. The main difference between the two lies in the quantity required and the roles they play in the body.

1. **Macronutrients:** Macronutrients are nutrients that are needed in larger quantities and provide energy (calories) to the body. There are three main macronutrients:

    a. **Carbohydrates:** Carbohydrates are the body's primary source of energy. They are broken down into glucose, which fuels bodily functions. Sources of carbohydrates include grains, fruits, vegetables, and legumes.

    b. **Proteins:** Proteins are essential for growth, repair, and maintenance of body tissues. They are made up of amino acids, which are the building blocks of proteins. Sources of proteins include meat, fish, dairy products, legumes, and nuts.

    c. **Fats:** Fats provide energy, support cell growth, and help absorb certain vitamins. They are essential for hormone production and insulation of organs. Sources of healthy fats include avocados, nuts, seeds, and oils like olive oil.

2. **Micronutrients:** Micronutrients are required in smaller amounts, but they are still vital for maintaining overall health. Micronutrients do not provide energy directly, but they play essential roles in various bodily functions. Micronutrients include vitamins and minerals:

   a. **Vitamins:** Vitamins are organic compounds that are required in small quantities for various bodily processes, such as metabolism, immune function, and tissue repair. Examples of vitamins include vitamin A, B vitamins, vitamin C, vitamin D, vitamin E, and vitamin K. They can be obtained from a balanced diet or supplements.

   b. **Minerals:** Minerals are inorganic substances required for normal body functioning, including building strong bones, transmitting nerve impulses, and maintaining fluid balance. Examples of minerals include calcium, iron, magnesium, potassium, and zinc. They can be obtained from a varied diet that includes fruits, vegetables, whole grains, and dairy products.

In summary, macronutrients are needed in larger quantities and provide energy, while micronutrients are required in smaller amounts and play crucial roles in various bodily functions. Both macronutrients and micronutrients are necessary for maintaining optimal health and well-being.

The Top Five Foundational Supplements You Should Consider Taking If You Are Near Fifty or Older

In this fast-paced world our bodies need a little extra help to stay functioning at our best. That's where vitamins come in. The give our body that extra boost to help you stay fit and feeling and looking younger.

First lest start with the disclaimer. This article is not intended to disburse medical advice. Everything is not for everybody. For example, while Vitamin K is not one of the top five, if you are on warfarin or other blood thinners you should not be taking vitamin K supplements. Consult your healthcare professional for medical advice.

These recommendations are based upon exhaustive research of scientific literature, peer reviewed articles, interviews with doctors researchers and professionals in the health supplement industry.

The Top Five Are:

1. Vitamin D3

2. Vitamin B3 (Niacinamide)

3. Curcumin

4. Hydrolyzed Collagen

5. CoQ 10

Briefly, Here's Why (in subsequent issues we will take a deeper dive into each of the top five)

1. Vitamin D works with calcium to support your bones and has also been shown to help strengthen muscles. It may play a role in regulating mood and protecting from viruses bacteria and respiratory tract infections. Studies have also shown that vitamin D helps fight inflammation and having adequate levels of Vitamin D may help prevent heart disease, stroke, high blood pressure and heart attacks.

2. Vitamin B3 also known as niacin plays a role in regulating good cholesterol by helping the body use proteins fats and converting food into energy. It helps maintain a healthy nervous system and is good for the skin and hair.

3. Curcumin, a natural STAT 3 inhibitor has been researched and may play a role in the prevention of certain cancers, Researchers are also looking into its role in delaying Alzheimer's, treating arthritis, and controlling diabetes

4. Hydrolyzed Collagen is one of the most researched supplements for shin health, skin elasticity and smoothing out wrinkles. Growing research has found that collagen helps to manage chronic joint pain,

skeletal muscular and is a great nutrient for the lining of the gut. Hydrolyzed Collagen has been broken down through the process of hydrolysis to make the is easier to be absorbed.

5. CoQ 10 decreases as we age. CoQ 10 has been shown to help improve the health of the heart while regulating blood sugar. It is said to also support prevention of periodontal disease, support brain and lung health and improve exercise performance.

You Can Find These Foundational Supplements In The YPL Store Click on Store: https://yourphenomenallife.net/store

What are the reported health effects of curcumin against cancer?

Curcumin, a compound found in the spice turmeric, has been extensively studied for its potential health benefits, including its effects on cancer. While research is ongoing and more studies are needed to fully understand the mechanisms and potential benefits, there is evidence to suggest that curcumin may have some anti-cancer properties. Here are some reported health effects of curcumin against cancer:

1. **Anti-inflammatory effects:** Curcumin has been found to exhibit strong anti-inflammatory properties. Chronic inflammation is linked to the development and progression of various types of cancer. By reducing inflammation, curcumin may help prevent the initiation and progression of cancer cells.

2. **Antioxidant activity:** Curcumin acts as a potent antioxidant, protecting cells from damage caused by free radicals. Free radicals can cause oxidative stress, which may contribute to the development of cancer. Curcumin's antioxidant activity may help neutralize these harmful molecules and prevent DNA damage.

3. **Inhibition of tumor growth:** Curcumin has been shown to inhibit the growth of various types of cancer cells in laboratory studies. It can interfere with multiple cellular signaling pathways involved in cancer development and progression, including those related to cell proliferation, apoptosis (cell death), angiogenesis (formation of new blood vessels), and metastasis (spread of cancer).

4. **Induction of apoptosis:** Curcumin has been reported to induce programmed cell death, or apoptosis, in cancer cells. Apoptosis is a natural process that helps eliminate damaged or abnormal cells. By promoting apoptosis in cancer cells, curcumin may help prevent tumor growth and progression.

5. **Modulation of gene expression:** Curcumin can influence the expression of genes involved in cancer development. It has been found to affect the activity of various genes related to cell cycle regulation, inflammation, metastasis, and angiogenesis. By modulating gene expression, curcumin may have a regulatory effect on cancer cells.

6. **Sensitization to chemotherapy and radiation:** Curcumin has been shown to enhance the effectiveness of certain chemotherapy drugs and radiation therapy in some studies. It may help sensitize cancer cells to these treatments, making them more susceptible to their effects. This could potentially improve treatment outcomes and reduce the resistance of cancer cells to therapy.

While these findings are promising, it's important to note that most studies have been conducted in laboratory settings or animal models, and more clinical trials are needed to determine the efficacy and safety of curcumin as a cancer treatment in humans. Curcumin supplements may also have limited bioavailability, meaning they are not well-absorbed by the body. Further research is underway to develop formulations that enhance curcumin's bioavailability and maximize its potential health benefits.

What are the health benefits of cranberry juice?

Cranberry juice is often praised for its potential health benefits. Here are some of the main benefits associated with consuming cranberry juice:

1. Urinary Tract Health: Cranberry juice has long been recognized for its ability to support urinary tract health. It contains compounds called proanthocyanidins, which may help prevent certain types of bacteria, particularly Escherichia coli (E. coli), from adhering to the urinary tract walls. This

action may reduce the risk of urinary tract infections (UTIs) and may be particularly beneficial for individuals prone to recurrent UTIs.

2. Antioxidant Properties: Cranberry juice is rich in antioxidants, such as vitamin C and various phytochemicals. Antioxidants help protect the body against damage caused by harmful free radicals, which can contribute to various diseases and the aging process. Regular consumption of cranberry juice may help reduce oxidative stress and inflammation in the body.

3. Heart Health: Some studies suggest that the antioxidants found in cranberry juice may have a positive impact on heart health. It may help lower blood pressure, reduce LDL (bad) cholesterol levels, and improve overall cardiovascular function. However, further research is needed to fully understand the extent of cranberry juice's effects on heart health.

4. Digestive Health: Cranberry juice contains dietary fiber, which can promote healthy digestion and prevent constipation. It may also have a mild laxative effect, helping to regulate bowel movements.

5. Oral Health: Cranberry juice may contribute to improved oral health. It may help prevent the bacteria responsible for tooth decay and gum disease from sticking to the teeth and gums. However, it's worth noting that cranberry juice is acidic, and excessive consumption may erode tooth enamel.

Therefore, it's important to consume it in moderation and practice good oral hygiene.

6. Anti-Inflammatory Effects: Some research suggests that the antioxidants and phytochemicals in cranberry juice have anti-inflammatory properties. This may be beneficial for conditions such as arthritis, cardiovascular disease, and certain types of cancer. However, more studies are needed to confirm these potential benefits.

It's important to note that while cranberry juice offers potential health benefits, it's often consumed in the form of sweetened and commercially processed beverages, which can be high in added sugars and calories. To maximize the health benefits, opt for unsweetened cranberry juice or consider incorporating whole cranberries into your diet. As always, it's a good idea to consult with a healthcare professional or registered dietitian for personalized advice and recommendations.

What is the benefit of beet juice in helping to control high blood pressure?

Beet juice has gained popularity for its potential benefits in helping to control high blood pressure, also known as hypertension. Heads Up! When I began using beet juice nobody told me that it will turn your urine red. I freaked out and thought I had blood in my urine. Here are some of the ways beet juice may contribute to blood pressure management:

1. **Nitric oxide production:** Beets are rich in dietary nitrates, which the body converts into nitric oxide. Nitric oxide acts as a vasodilator, meaning it relaxes and widens blood vessels, promoting improved blood flow and reduced pressure on arterial walls.

2. **Lowered peripheral resistance:** By dilating blood vessels, beet juice may help lower peripheral resistance, which refers to the resistance the blood encounters as it flows through the small blood vessels. Reduced resistance can lead to a decrease in blood pressure.

3. **Antioxidant properties:** Beets contain antioxidants, such as betalains, that help reduce oxidative stress and inflammation in the body. This may positively influence blood pressure levels, as oxidative stress and inflammation can contribute to hypertension.

4. **Potential anti-inflammatory effects:** Chronic inflammation can contribute to high blood

pressure. Some research suggests that beet juice may have anti-inflammatory effects, which could indirectly help in managing blood pressure.

5. **Natural source of potassium**: Beets are a good source of potassium, a mineral that plays a vital role in maintaining healthy blood pressure. Adequate potassium intake is associated with reduced blood pressure levels.

While beet juice may offer benefits for blood pressure management, it is important to note that individual results may vary, and it should not replace medical advice or prescribed medications. If you have hypertension, it's crucial to consult with your healthcare provider to determine the best course of action for managing your blood pressure.

What is hydrolyzed collagen, and does it work?

Hydrolyzed collagen, also known as collagen peptides, has gained popularity as a supplement in recent years. Collagen is a protein found in our bodies, particularly in the skin, bones, tendons, and ligaments, and it provides structural support and elasticity to these tissues.

Hydrolyzed collagen is produced by breaking down collagen molecules into smaller peptides, making it easier for the body to absorb and utilize. The theory behind taking hydrolyzed collagen supplements is that they can promote collagen production in the body, potentially benefiting the health and appearance of the skin, hair, nails, and joints.

While there is some evidence suggesting that hydrolyzed collagen may have certain benefits, it's important to note that more research is needed to establish its effectiveness and understand its mechanisms of action fully. Some studies have shown positive results, while others have been inconclusive.

Here are a few potential benefits of hydrolyzed collagen that have been suggested by preliminary research:

1. **Skin health:** Some studies have found that taking hydrolyzed collagen supplements may help improve skin elasticity, hydration, and reduce the appearance of wrinkles. However, the evidence is limited, and more research is needed to confirm these findings.

2. **Joint health:** Collagen is a vital component of cartilage, which cushions and supports joints. Some studies have indicated that hydrolyzed collagen might help reduce joint pain and improve joint function in people with osteoarthritis. However, the evidence is mixed, and further research is required.

3. **Nail and hair health:** Collagen is a significant component of nails and hair, and some anecdotal reports suggest that hydrolyzed collagen supplements can help strengthen nails and promote hair growth. However, scientific evidence supporting these claims is lacking.

It's important to note that collagen supplements, including hydrolyzed collagen, are not regulated by the U.S. Food and Drug Administration (FDA) in the same way as pharmaceutical drugs. Therefore, the quality and efficacy of these supplements can vary. If you are considering taking hydrolyzed collagen or any other supplement, it's best to consult with a healthcare professional who can provide personalized advice based on your specific needs and health conditions.

What is Fo Ti

Fo ti, also known as He Shou Wu or Polygonum multiflorum, is a traditional Chinese herb that has been used for centuries in traditional medicine. It is a perennial vine native to China and is also found in other parts of Asia.

The herb is derived from the root of the plant and is commonly used for its potential health benefits. It is believed to possess adaptogenic properties, meaning it may help the body cope with stress and promote overall well-being. Fo ti is also known for its reputed anti-aging effects and is often used to support healthy aging and promote longevity.

In traditional Chinese medicine, fo ti is used to nourish the liver and kidneys, as well as to invigorate the blood and promote circulation. It is also believed to support healthy hair growth and help maintain the health of the skin.

Fo ti is available in various forms, including capsules, powders, and liquid extracts. It can be consumed internally as a dietary supplement or used externally in hair care products or topical applications.

It's important to note that while Fo Ti has a long history of use in traditional medicine, scientific research on its effectiveness and safety is limited. If you are considering using fo ti as a dietary supplement or for any health-related purposes, it is advisable to consult with a healthcare professional or a qualified herbalist to determine the appropriate dosage and to discuss any potential risks or interactions with other medications or conditions.

What is balloon flower used for ?

Balloon flower, scientifically known as Platycodon important as, is a perennial plant native to East Asia. It is primarily cultivated for its attractive flowers and is a popular choice in gardens and landscapes. However, beyond its ornamental value, balloon flower has a few uses:

1. **Medicinal Purposes:** In traditional Asian medicine, various parts of the balloon flower plant, including the root, are used for their potential health benefits. It is believed to possess anti-inflammatory, antibacterial, and expectorant properties. Balloon flower root is commonly used in herbal remedies for respiratory conditions like coughs, colds, and bronchitis.

2. **Culinary Applications:** In some Asian cuisines, the young shoots and roots of the balloon flower plant are consumed as vegetables. The tender shoots can be stir-fried, added to soups, or used in salads. The root is often used in traditional Korean cuisine and is known as "doraji."

3. **Ornamental Value:** As mentioned earlier, balloon flower is primarily cultivated for its appealing flowers. The flowers are balloon-shaped buds that open into star-shaped blossoms in various shades of blue, purple, pink, or white. Balloon flowers add beauty to gardens, flower beds, and borders.

It's worth noting that while balloon flower has historical and cultural uses, the effectiveness of its medicinal properties and safety for consumption should be approached with caution. It's always advisable to consult with a healthcare professional or an expert in herbal medicine before using any plant for medicinal purposes.

In Chinese herbal medicine what is spring wine?

In traditional Chinese herbal medicine, "spring wine" refers to a type of medicinal wine that is typically made by infusing herbs and other ingredients in alcohol. It is commonly consumed during the spring season as part of traditional health practices.

Spring wine is believed to have invigorating and nourishing properties that help to promote vitality and balance in the body. The specific herbs and ingredients used can vary depending on the desired therapeutic effects. Some commonly used herbs in Chinese spring wines include ginseng, astragalus, goji berries, Chinese dates, and various other medicinal plants.

These herbal ingredients are typically soaked or steeped in a high-proof alcohol, such as rice wine or grain alcohol, for a period of time to extract their beneficial properties. The resulting wine is then consumed in small amounts, often as a tonic or as a part of a larger herbal regimen.

It's important to note that the use of herbal medicines, including spring wines, should be done under the guidance of a qualified practitioner of traditional Chinese medicine, as they can have interactions with medications and may not be suitable for everyone.

What is ginseng used for?

Ginseng is a popular medicinal herb that has been used for centuries in traditional medicine systems, particularly in East Asia. It is derived from the roots of plants belonging to the Panax genus, such as Panax ginseng (Asian ginseng) and Panax quinquefolius (American ginseng).

Ginseng is known for its adaptogenic properties, which means it may help the body cope with physical and mental stressors. It contains active compounds called ginsenosides, which are believed to be responsible for its medicinal effects. Here are some common uses of ginseng:

1. **Boosting energy and reducing fatigue:** Ginseng is often used to increase energy levels and combat fatigue. It is believed to have stimulating effects on the central nervous system, helping to improve physical and mental performance.

2. **Enhancing cognitive function:** Ginseng has been traditionally used to improve memory, concentration, and overall cognitive function. Some studies suggest that it may have neuroprotective properties and could potentially benefit individuals with cognitive decline or neurodegenerative diseases.

3. **Supporting immune health:** Ginseng has been associated with immune-boosting properties. It may help strengthen the immune system, making the body more resistant to infections and diseases.

4. **Improving physical stamina and endurance:** Athletes and fitness enthusiasts often use ginseng to enhance their physical performance. It is believed to improve endurance, increase oxygen uptake, and reduce recovery time after exercise.

5. **Managing stress and promoting relaxation:** Ginseng is considered an adaptogen, which means it may help the body adapt to and manage stress. It is believed to have a calming effect and may help reduce anxiety and improve overall well-being.

6. **Supporting sexual health:** Ginseng has been traditionally used as an aphrodisiac and to improve sexual function in both men and women. Some studies suggest that ginseng may enhance sexual desire, improve erectile function, and alleviate symptoms of menopause.

It's important to note that while ginseng has a long history of use and many potential health benefits, scientific research is still ongoing to fully understand its effects and mechanisms of action. As with any herbal supplement, it's advisable to consult with a healthcare professional before using ginseng, especially if you have any underlying health conditions or are taking other medications.

What is dong quai?

"Dong Quai" (also known as "Angelica sinensis") is an herb that is native to China, Japan, and Korea. It has been used for centuries in traditional Chinese medicine as a remedy for various health conditions. Dong Quai is particularly renowned for its potential benefits in women's health.

Dong Quai is often referred to as the "female ginseng" due to its historical use as a tonic for women. It is commonly used to help regulate menstrual cycles and relieve symptoms associated with menstruation, such as cramps and mood swings. Some women also use Dong Quai to alleviate symptoms of menopause, such as hot flashes and vaginal dryness.

Additionally, Dong Quai is believed to have blood-thinning properties and may enhance blood circulation. It is sometimes used to alleviate symptoms of poor circulation, such as cold hands and feet. However, it's important to note that more scientific research is needed to fully understand and confirm the benefits of Dong Quai.

As with any herbal supplement, it's crucial to consult with a healthcare professional before using Dong Quai, especially if you have any underlying medical conditions or are taking other medications. They can provide personalized advice based on your specific situation and guide you on the appropriate dosage and potential interactions.

What is Dit Da Jow?

Dit da jow, also known as dit da jiu or dit da zhou, is a traditional Chinese liniment used in martial arts and traditional Chinese medicine. The name "dit da jow" roughly translates to "fall and hit wine" or "hit-fall wine" in English. It is a topical herbal formula that is applied externally to the body to help promote healing and alleviate pain associated with injuries, bruises, sprains, and strains.

The exact formulation of dit da jow can vary depending on the specific recipe or lineage, but it typically consists of a combination of Chinese herbs, roots, barks, and sometimes animal products. Common ingredients include herbs such as arnica, myrrh, frankincense, dragon's blood, safflower, cinnamon, and various other botanicals. These ingredients are usually soaked in a base of alcohol, such as rice wine or medicinal alcohol, to extract their medicinal properties.

Dit da jow is believed to work by improving blood circulation, reducing inflammation, and promoting the healing of damaged tissues. It is commonly used by martial artists, especially those practicing Chinese martial arts like kung fu, to aid in injury prevention, speed up recovery, and alleviate pain associated with training or combat-related injuries. It is often applied through massage or by soaking a cloth or cotton ball in the liniment and then applying it to the affected area.

It's worth noting that while dit da jow has been used for centuries in Chinese medicine and martial arts, its effectiveness and specific benefits have not been extensively studied or validated by modern scientific research. It is primarily regarded as a traditional remedy and is often passed down through generations within martial arts lineages. As with any herbal remedy or medicinal product, it is advisable to consult with a qualified healthcare professional before using dit da jow, especially if you have any pre-existing medical conditions or are taking medications.

What are the benefits of resveratrol supplements?

Resveratrol is a natural compound found in certain foods and beverages, particularly in red wine, grapes, and berries. It has gained attention due to its potential health benefits. While more research is needed to fully understand its effects, here are some of the potential benefits of resveratrol supplementation:

1. **Antioxidant properties:** Resveratrol is known for its antioxidant activity, which helps protect cells from damage caused by harmful free radicals. Antioxidants are important for maintaining overall health and reducing the risk of chronic diseases.

2. **Anti-inflammatory effects:** Resveratrol has been shown to possess anti-inflammatory properties, which may help reduce inflammation in the body. Chronic inflammation is associated with various health conditions, including cardiovascular disease, diabetes, and certain types of cancer.

3. **Cardiovascular health:** Resveratrol has been studied for its potential benefits in promoting cardiovascular health. It may help improve blood flow, reduce blood clot formation, lower blood pressure, and increase the levels of "good" HDL cholesterol while reducing "bad" LDL cholesterol.

4. **Brain health:** Some studies suggest that resveratrol may have neuroprotective properties and could potentially play a role in supporting brain health. It has been investigated for its potential to enhance cognitive function and protect against age-related neurodegenerative diseases such as Alzheimer's and Parkinson's disease.

5. **Anti-aging effects:** Resveratrol has been associated with potential anti-aging effects. It may activate certain genes and enzymes involved in cellular longevity and enhance the function of mitochondria, the powerhouses of cells.

6. **Potential cancer prevention:** Resveratrol has shown promise in laboratory studies as a potential anticancer agent. It has been observed to inhibit the growth of cancer cells and induce apoptosis

(programmed cell death). However, more research is needed to determine its effectiveness in humans.

It's important to note that while resveratrol has demonstrated these potential benefits in laboratory and animal studies, the evidence in humans is limited and sometimes conflicting. The bioavailability of resveratrol from dietary sources is relatively low, and it can be challenging to achieve therapeutic levels through supplementation alone. Additionally, individual responses to resveratrol supplementation may vary. As with any supplement, it's advisable to consult with a healthcare professional before starting resveratrol or any other dietary supplement to determine its suitability for your specific needs and health conditions.

What are the benefits of Pterostilbene supplementation?

Pterostilbene is a natural compound found in certain plants, including blueberries and grapes. It belongs to a class of compounds called stilbenoids, which are known for their antioxidant and anti-inflammatory properties. Pterostilbene has gained attention in the field of nutrition and health due to its potential benefits. Here are some of the reported benefits of pterostilbene supplementation:

1. **Antioxidant activity:** Pterostilbene is a potent antioxidant, which means it helps protect cells from oxidative stress caused by free radicals. This antioxidant activity may have various positive effects on health, including reducing the risk of

chronic diseases such as cardiovascular disease, neurodegenerative disorders, and cancer.

2. **Anti-inflammatory effects:** Pterostilbene has been found to possess anti-inflammatory properties. Chronic inflammation is associated with several health conditions, including heart disease, diabetes, and certain cancers. By reducing inflammation, pterostilbene may help promote overall health and potentially reduce the risk of these diseases.

3. **Cardiovascular health:** Pterostilbene has been studied for its potential cardiovascular benefits. It has been shown to help lower blood pressure, reduce LDL cholesterol levels, and inhibit the formation of plaques in the arteries. These effects may contribute to a reduced risk of heart disease and improved cardiovascular health.

4. **Cognitive function:** Some research suggests that pterostilbene may have positive effects on cognitive function and brain health. It has been found to exhibit neuroprotective properties, potentially protecting against age-related cognitive decline and neurodegenerative disorders such as Alzheimer's disease.

5. **Blood sugar control:** Pterostilbene may have a positive impact on blood sugar control. It has been found to improve insulin sensitivity and enhance glucose metabolism, which can help regulate blood sugar levels. This potential benefit may be

particularly relevant for individuals with diabetes or those at risk of developing the condition.

6. **Weight management:** Preliminary studies have suggested that pterostilbene may help support healthy weight management. It has been found to influence lipid metabolism, promote fat burning, and inhibit fat storage in animal studies. However, further research is needed to better understand its effects on human weight management.

It's important to note that while there is promising research on pterostilbene's potential benefits, many studies have been conducted in animals or in vitro (in a laboratory setting). More research is needed to fully understand the effects and potential applications of pterostilbene in humans. If you're considering pterostilbene supplementation, it's recommended to consult with a healthcare professional for personalized advice and guidance.

As we age what is the importance of Vitamin D?

Vitamin D plays a crucial role in our overall health as we age. Here are some important aspects of vitamin D and its significance:

1. **Bone Health:** Vitamin D helps regulate calcium and phosphorus levels in the body, which are essential for maintaining strong and healthy bones. It aids in the absorption of calcium from the intestines and promotes its deposition in bones, thereby reducing

the risk of fractures and osteoporosis, a condition characterized by weakened bones.

2. **Muscle Function:** Adequate vitamin D levels are important for optimal muscle function and strength, particularly in older adults. Deficiency in vitamin D has been linked to muscle weakness, balance problems, and an increased risk of falls and fractures.

3. **Immune System Support:** Vitamin D plays a crucial role in modulating the immune system. It helps regulate immune cell function and supports the body's defense against infections and diseases. As we age, our immune system may weaken, making vitamin D even more important for maintaining a healthy immune response.

4. **Heart Health:** Vitamin D deficiency has been associated with an increased risk of cardiovascular diseases, including hypertension, heart attacks, and strokes. Adequate levels of vitamin D may help promote cardiovascular health and reduce the risk of these conditions.

5. **Cognitive Function:** Some research suggests a potential link between vitamin D deficiency and cognitive decline in older adults. Maintaining sufficient vitamin D levels may help support cognitive function and reduce the risk of conditions such as dementia and Alzheimer's disease.

6. **Mood and Mental Health:** Low vitamin D levels have been associated with an increased risk of depression, particularly in older adults. Adequate vitamin D levels may contribute to better mood and mental well-being.

It's worth noting that while vitamin D can be synthesized by the body when exposed to sunlight, as we age, our skin's ability to produce vitamin D decreases. Additionally, factors such as reduced outdoor activities, limited sun exposure, and certain health conditions can contribute to vitamin D deficiency in older adults. Therefore, it is important to maintain appropriate vitamin D levels through a combination of sunlight exposure, diet, and potentially supplementation, under the guidance of a healthcare professional.

What is Co Q 10

Coenzyme Q10, commonly known as CoQ10, is a naturally occurring compound found in every cell of the human body. It plays a vital role in cellular energy production and acts as an antioxidant to protect cells from damage. CoQ10 is also known as ubiquinone because it is ubiquitous (found everywhere) in the body.

CoQ10 is involved in the electron transport chain, a process that occurs within the mitochondria of cells, where it helps convert food into adenosine triphosphate (ATP), the molecule that provides energy for cellular activities. As an antioxidant, CoQ10 helps neutralize harmful free radicals, which are unstable molecules that can cause oxidative damage to cells.

While the body can produce CoQ10 naturally, its production may decline with age or due to certain medical conditions. Additionally, some medications, such as cholesterol-lowering statins, can lower CoQ10 levels in the body. In such cases, CoQ10 supplements may be used to replenish the levels.

CoQ10 supplements are available in various forms, including capsules, tablets, and softgels. It is important to note that CoQ10 is a fat-soluble compound, so it is often recommended to take it with a meal that contains some fat to enhance absorption.

Research suggests that CoQ10 may have potential benefits for several health conditions, such as heart disease, high blood pressure, migraines, and certain neurological disorders. However, more studies are needed to fully understand its effectiveness and determine appropriate dosages for specific conditions.

As with any supplement, it is recommended to consult with a healthcare professional before starting CoQ10 supplementation to discuss potential benefits, proper dosage, and any potential interactions with medications or existing health conditions.

What are the healing properties of Sour Sop?

Soursop, also known as Graviola or Guanabana, is a tropical fruit native to the Americas. While there is limited scientific research on the specific healing properties of soursop, it is believed to offer several potential health benefits. However, it's important to note that these claims are based on traditional usage and anecdotal evidence, and further scientific studies are needed to fully understand its effects.

Here are some of the potential healing properties associated with soursop:

1. **Antioxidant properties:** Soursop is rich in antioxidants, such as vitamin C, which helps protect the body's cells from damage caused by free radicals.

2. **Immune system support:** The fruit contains various compounds that may support immune function, including antioxidants and vitamin C. A healthy immune system is vital for overall well-being.

3. **Anti-inflammatory effects:** Soursop may possess anti-inflammatory properties, which can help reduce inflammation in the body. Chronic inflammation is associated with various health conditions and reducing it may promote better health.

4. **Digestive health:** Soursop is often used to promote digestive health and relieve gastrointestinal issues. It may have mild laxative properties and can be used to alleviate constipation.

5. **Potential anti-cancer properties:** Some preliminary studies suggest that soursop may contain compounds with anti-cancer effects. However, more research is needed to determine the effectiveness and safety of soursop as a treatment for cancer.

6. **Antimicrobial activity:** Soursop has been traditionally used in some cultures to treat infections and as a natural remedy for parasites due to its potential antimicrobial properties.

It's important to note that while soursop shows promise for its potential health benefits, it is not a substitute for medical treatment. If you have any specific health concerns, it is always best to consult with a healthcare professional for proper diagnosis and treatment.

What are the healing properties of Oregano Oil?

Oregano oil is derived from the leaves and flowers of the oregano plant, scientifically known as Origanum vulgare. It has been used for centuries in traditional medicine for its potential healing properties. While it's important to note that scientific research is still ongoing and further studies are needed to fully understand its effects, here are some potential healing properties associated with oregano oil:

1. **Antibacterial and antifungal properties:** Oregano oil contains compounds such as carvacrol and thymol, which have shown antimicrobial activity against various bacteria and fungi. It may be used to help fight off infections caused by these microorganisms.

2. **Antiviral properties:** Some studies suggest that oregano oil may have antiviral effects and could potentially help inhibit the growth of certain viruses. However, more research is needed in this area.

3. **Anti-inflammatory effects:** Oregano oil contains components that possess anti-inflammatory properties. It may help reduce inflammation and alleviate associated symptoms, although its specific mechanisms are not yet fully understood.

4. **Digestive support:** Oregano oil has been used traditionally to aid digestion and relieve symptoms such as bloating, gas, and indigestion. It may also possess mild laxative properties.

5. **Antioxidant activity:** The antioxidants present in oregano oil, such as rosmarinic acid and thymol, may help protect cells against oxidative damage caused by free radicals.

6. **Respiratory support:** Oregano oil is commonly used as a natural remedy for respiratory conditions, such as coughs, colds, and sinus infections. It may help relieve congestion and soothe throat discomfort.

7. **Skin health:** Topical application of diluted oregano oil may offer benefits for certain skin conditions, including acne, fungal infections, and insect bites. However, it should always be used with caution and properly diluted to avoid skin irritation.

It's worth mentioning that oregano oil is highly concentrated and using it in excessive amounts or undiluted form can cause skin irritation, digestive upset, or other adverse effects. It's important to consult with a healthcare professional or a qualified herbalist before using oregano oil for therapeutic purposes, especially if you have any pre-existing medical conditions or are taking medications.

What are the healing properties of Deer Antler?

Deer antler has been used in traditional Chinese medicine for centuries due to its perceived healing properties. However, it's important to note that the scientific evidence supporting these claims is limited, and more research is needed to fully understand the effects of deer antler on human health. Here are some of the commonly attributed healing properties:

1. **Joint Health:** Deer antler velvet is often marketed as a remedy for joint pain and inflammation. It is believed to contain substances that promote the growth and repair of cartilage, potentially benefiting conditions like osteoarthritis. However, studies on its effectiveness have shown mixed results.

2. **Athletic Performance and Recovery:** Some athletes and bodybuilders use deer antler supplements, claiming they can enhance strength, endurance, and muscle recovery. These claims are based on the presence of insulin-like growth factor 1 (IGF-1) in deer antler velvet, which is believed to stimulate

muscle growth. However, evidence supporting these claims is currently lacking.

3. **Sexual Health:** Deer antler is also believed to have aphrodisiac properties and may be used to improve sexual function and fertility. However, there is insufficient scientific evidence to confirm these effects.

4. **Immune System Support:** Some traditional uses of deer antler include boosting the immune system and increasing resistance to illness. However, more research is needed to understand its impact on immune function.

5. **Anti-aging Effects:** Deer antler is sometimes promoted for its potential anti-aging properties, such as improving skin health and reducing wrinkles. However, scientific evidence supporting these claims is lacking.

It's crucial to consult with a qualified healthcare professional before using deer antler products, as they may interact with medications or have side effects. Additionally, be cautious when purchasing deer antler products, as the market is largely unregulated, and the quality and purity of these supplements can vary significantly.

Green Tea

Green tea has been widely studied for its medicinal properties and is known for its potential health benefits. Here are some of the medicinal properties associated with green tea:

1. **Antioxidant effects:** Green tea is rich in antioxidants, particularly catechins such as epigallocatechin gallate (EGCG). These antioxidants help protect cells from damage caused by free radicals, which are unstable molecules associated with various diseases and aging processes.

2. **Anti-inflammatory properties:** Green tea contains compounds that have anti-inflammatory effects. Regular consumption of green tea has been associated with a reduced risk of chronic inflammatory conditions such as arthritis and cardiovascular diseases.

3. **Heart health:** Green tea has been linked to improvements in cardiovascular health. It may help reduce LDL cholesterol levels (the "bad" cholesterol) and triglycerides, and improve overall cholesterol profiles. Green tea consumption has also been associated with a reduced risk of developing heart disease.

4. **Weight management:** Green tea has been studied for its potential role in weight management. It contains compounds that can help boost metabolism and increase fat oxidation. Some studies suggest that

green tea extract may aid in weight loss and fat reduction.

5. **Diabetes management:** Green tea consumption has been associated with a lower risk of developing type 2 diabetes. It may help regulate blood sugar levels and improve insulin sensitivity. Green tea may also contribute to weight management, which is important in preventing and managing diabetes.

6. **Cancer prevention:** Some research suggests that the antioxidants in green tea may help protect against certain types of cancers, such as breast, prostate, and colorectal cancers. However, more studies are needed to fully understand the effects of green tea on cancer prevention and treatment.

7. **Brain health:** Green tea contains caffeine and an amino acid called L-theanine, which may have beneficial effects on brain function. The combination of caffeine and L-theanine can improve focus, attention, and alertness. Green tea consumption has also been associated with a reduced risk of neurodegenerative diseases like Alzheimer's and Parkinson's.

8. **Dental health:** The antibacterial properties of green tea can help inhibit the growth of oral bacteria and reduce the risk of dental cavities, gum disease, and bad breath. Some toothpaste and mouthwash products contain green tea extracts for these reasons.

It's important to note that while green tea has potential health benefits, individual results may vary, and it should not be considered a cure-all for any condition. It's always recommended to consult with a healthcare professional for personalized advice and guidance.

What are the medicinal benefits of Ginko Bioloba?

Ginkgo biloba, commonly known as ginkgo or maidenhair tree, is a unique tree species native to China. It has been used for centuries in traditional Chinese medicine for various purposes. While some people believe in its medicinal benefits, it's important to note that scientific research on ginkgo biloba has yielded mixed results, and the U.S. Food and Drug Administration (FDA) does not approve it as a drug for treating any specific medical conditions. However, here are some of the potential medicinal benefits that have been studied:

1. **Cognitive function:** Ginkgo biloba has been investigated for its potential to improve cognitive function and memory in conditions such as Alzheimer's disease, dementia, and age-related cognitive decline. Some studies have suggested that ginkgo biloba extract may have a modest positive effect on memory and cognition, although the results have been inconsistent.

2. **Antioxidant properties:** Ginkgo biloba contains compounds with antioxidant properties, which means they can help neutralize harmful free radicals

in the body. Antioxidants are believed to protect cells from oxidative stress and damage. This property of ginkgo biloba extract may have potential benefits for overall health and well-being.

3. **Peripheral circulation:** Ginkgo biloba has been studied for its potential to improve blood flow and circulation, particularly in the peripheral areas of the body. It may help dilate blood vessels, reduce blood clotting, and improve oxygen supply to tissues. Some people use ginkgo biloba to alleviate symptoms associated with poor circulation, such as leg pain, cold hands and feet, and tinnitus (ringing in the ears).

4. **Eye health:** Some research suggests that ginkgo biloba extract may have a positive impact on certain eye conditions. It has been investigated for its potential to improve vision in people with glaucoma, diabetic retinopathy, and age-related macular degeneration (AMD). However, more research is needed to establish its effectiveness in these specific conditions.

5. **Anxiety and depression:** Ginkgo biloba has been used traditionally for its potential mood-enhancing effects. Some studies have explored its use as an adjunctive therapy for anxiety and depression. However, the evidence is limited and conflicting, and more rigorous research is required.

It's important to consult with a healthcare professional before using ginkgo biloba or any herbal supplement, especially if you have underlying medical conditions, take medications, or are pregnant or breastfeeding. They can provide personalized advice based on your specific circumstances.

What are the benefits of Royal Jelly?

Royal jelly is a nutritious substance produced by worker bees to feed and nurture the queen bee throughout her life. It is highly regarded for its potential health benefits and has been used in traditional medicine for centuries. While scientific research on royal jelly is still ongoing, here are some of the potential benefits associated with its consumption:

1. **Nutritional value:** Royal jelly is rich in proteins, vitamins (B-complex vitamins, vitamin C, and vitamin E), minerals (such as calcium, magnesium, and potassium), essential amino acids, and fatty acids. It can provide a natural boost of nutrition when consumed.

2. **Antioxidant properties:** Royal jelly contains antioxidants that help combat oxidative stress in the body. Antioxidants help neutralize harmful free radicals, which are associated with various diseases and aging.

3. **Anti-inflammatory effects:** Some studies suggest that royal jelly may possess anti-inflammatory properties. It has been found to inhibit the production of pro-inflammatory compounds, potentially helping to reduce inflammation in the body.

4. **Immune system support:** Royal jelly contains several compounds that may boost the immune system, such as proteins and peptides with antimicrobial properties. It may help enhance the body's natural defense mechanisms and protect against certain infections.

5. **Potential hormonal effects:** Royal jelly contains substances that may affect hormone levels in the body. It has been suggested to have estrogenic properties, potentially benefiting women during menopause or those experiencing hormonal imbalances.

6. **Skin health:** Due to its nutrient content and potential antioxidant properties, royal jelly is sometimes used in skincare products. It may help promote skin health, improve moisture retention, and contribute to a youthful appearance.

It's important to note that while royal jelly shows promise, more research is needed to fully understand its effects and determine its safety profile. Additionally, individuals who are allergic to bee products should avoid consuming royal jelly, as it can cause severe allergic reactions. If you have any specific health concerns, it's always recommended to consult with a healthcare professional before adding royal jelly or any other supplement to your routine.

What is a Sugar Detox?

A sugar detox involves reducing or eliminating added sugars from your diet for a specific period to reset your taste buds, stabilize blood sugar levels, and potentially break free from sugar cravings. Here are some steps to help you embark on a sugar detox:

1. **Set a clear goal:** Decide on the duration of your sugar detox and define what you want to achieve from the process. Having a clear goal will help you stay motivated and focused throughout the detox.

2. **Educate yourself:** Learn about different types of sugars, where they hide in food products, and how they can affect your health. This knowledge will help you make informed choices during the detox.

3. **Read labels:** Start reading food labels to identify hidden sugars. Keep an eye out for various sugar names, such as sucrose, high-fructose corn syrup, dextrose, maltose, and others.

4. **Gradually reduce sugar intake:** If you are used to consuming a lot of sugary foods and beverages, suddenly cutting them out can lead to withdrawal symptoms and make it challenging to stick to the detox. Gradually reduce your sugar intake over a few days or a week before beginning the detox.

5. **Clean out your pantry:** Get rid of sugary snacks, sweets, sugary beverages, and processed foods with high sugar content. Replace them with healthier

alternatives like fresh fruits, vegetables, nuts, and seeds.

6. **Plan your meals:** Create a meal plan that focuses on whole foods, such as lean proteins, vegetables, whole grains, and healthy fats. This will help you avoid processed foods that often contain added sugars.

7. **Stay hydrated:** Drink plenty of water throughout the day. Sometimes, our bodies can mistake thirst for hunger, leading to cravings for sugary snacks.

8. **Avoid artificial sweeteners:** While they may contain fewer or no calories, using artificial sweeteners during a sugar detox may perpetuate your desire for sweet tastes and hinder the reset of your taste buds.

9. **Choose healthy snacks:** When you feel the urge to snack, opt for healthy choices like fresh fruits, nuts, plain yogurt, or vegetables with hummus.

10. **Be mindful of condiments and sauces:** Many condiments and sauces contain hidden sugars. Choose options with little to no added sugars or make your own at home.

11. **Get enough sleep and manage stress:** Lack of sleep and stress can lead to sugar cravings. Ensure you get enough rest and practice stress-reducing activities like meditation or yoga.

12. **Track your progress: Keep** a journal or use a mobile app to track your daily food intake and note any changes in your energy levels, mood, and cravings.

Remember, a sugar detox is a short-term approach to reset your eating habits. After the detox, consider incorporating moderate amounts of natural sugars from whole foods back into your diet while still avoiding added sugars and highly processed foods as much as possible. Always consult with a healthcare professional before making significant changes to your diet, especially if you have any underlying health conditions.

What happens to the body during a sugar detox?

During a sugar detox, when you significantly reduce or eliminate added sugars from your diet, several changes can occur in the body as it adapts to the new dietary pattern. Here are some of the common things that happen during a sugar detox:

1. **Improved blood sugar levels:** By cutting out added sugars, your blood sugar levels become more stable. This can reduce fluctuations in energy levels and decrease the risk of insulin resistance, a precursor to type 2 diabetes.

2. **Reduced cravings:** As you break free from the cycle of consuming sugary foods, your taste buds gradually adapt to the lower sweetness level. This can lead to a reduced desire for sugary treats over time.

3. **Weight loss:** High-sugar diets are often associated with excessive calorie intake and weight gain. A sugar detox can lead to weight loss if you replace

sugary foods with healthier options and reduce overall calorie intake.

4. **Improved energy levels:** Relying on sugary foods for energy can lead to energy crashes and fatigue. During a sugar detox, as your blood sugar stabilizes, you may experience more consistent energy levels throughout the day.

5. **Better focus and mental clarity:** Some people report improved mental clarity and focus when they reduce sugar intake, as they are no longer experiencing sugar-induced energy spikes and crashes.

6. **Enhanced digestion:** High sugar consumption, especially from processed foods, can disrupt the balance of gut bacteria. Reducing sugar intake may support a healthier gut environment.

7. **Possible withdrawal symptoms:** When you stop consuming sugars abruptly, you might experience withdrawal symptoms, including headaches, irritability, mood swings, and cravings. These symptoms are temporary and usually subside within a few days.

8. **Reduced inflammation:** High sugar intake can contribute to inflammation in the body, which is linked to various chronic health conditions. Cutting back on sugar may help reduce inflammation levels.

9. **Better skin health:** Sugar can contribute to skin issues like acne and premature aging. Eliminating or reducing sugar intake may lead to clearer and healthier-looking skin.

10. **Lower risk of chronic diseases:** High sugar consumption is associated with an increased risk of obesity, type 2 diabetes, heart disease, and other chronic health conditions. A sugar detox can help lower these risks by promoting a healthier diet.

It's important to note that everyone's body responds differently to a sugar detox. Some people may experience these changes more dramatically than others. Additionally, if you have underlying health conditions or concerns, it's essential to consult with a healthcare professional before starting any significant dietary changes. A sugar detox is typically a short-term approach, and after the detox period, it's essential to adopt a balanced and sustainable eating plan that includes moderate amounts of natural sugars from whole foods while still minimizing added sugars and highly processed foods.

What exercises should be done after a stroke

After a stroke, it's essential to engage in a rehabilitation program tailored to the individual's specific needs and capabilities. The exercises should focus on improving physical and cognitive functions, enhancing balance, coordination, strength, and flexibility. Here are some common exercises that may be included in a post-stroke rehabilitation program:

1. **Range of motion exercises:** These exercises aim to improve flexibility and prevent muscle stiffness. They involve gentle movements of the affected limbs and joints.

2. **Strengthening exercises:** Targeting weak muscles can help regain strength and functional abilities. These exercises can include resistance training with weights or resistance bands.

3. **Balance and coordination exercises:** Post-stroke, balance and coordination may be affected. Exercises like standing on one leg, weight shifting, and walking on uneven surfaces can be beneficial.

4. **Walking exercises:** Gradual walking practice can help improve gait and walking abilities. This may involve assistance from therapists or assistive devices like canes or walkers.

5. **Functional activities:** Incorporating daily life activities into the rehabilitation process can help regain independence and confidence. These activities may include dressing, eating, and grooming tasks.

6. **Fine motor exercises:** To improve hand dexterity and fine motor skills, activities like picking up small objects, writing, or manipulating buttons can be incorporated.

7. **Cognitive exercises:** Stroke may affect cognitive functions such as memory, attention, and problem-

solving. Cognitive training activities can help address these challenges.

8. **Speech and language exercises:** For individuals with speech difficulties after a stroke, speech therapy can be beneficial in improving communication skills.

9. **Aquatic therapy:** Water-based exercises can be less taxing on the joints and provide a supportive environment for movement practice.

It's crucial to work with a qualified healthcare professional, such as a physical therapist, occupational therapist, or speech therapist, to design a personalized rehabilitation plan. The exercises and intensity will depend on the severity of the stroke and the individual's overall health and progress. Regularity and consistency in performing these exercises will aid in achieving the best possible recovery outcome.

What exercise is best for a person with diabetes?

For individuals with diabetes, it is essential to engage in regular physical activity as it can have numerous health benefits, including improved blood sugar control, weight management, increased insulin sensitivity, and reduced risk of cardiovascular complications. However, the best exercise for a person with diabetes can vary depending on their individual health status, fitness level, and personal preferences. Before starting any exercise program, it's crucial to consult with a healthcare professional or a certified diabetes educator to create a personalized plan that suits your specific needs.

That being said, some exercises generally considered beneficial for people with diabetes include:

1. **Aerobic exercises:** Activities that get your heart pumping and increase your breathing rate can help lower blood sugar levels and improve cardiovascular health. Examples include brisk walking, cycling, swimming, dancing, and jogging.

2. **Strength training:** Resistance exercises, such as weightlifting or bodyweight exercises, can help increase muscle mass and improve insulin sensitivity. Stronger muscles can also support joint health and help manage weight.

3. **Flexibility exercises:** Stretching exercises like yoga or tai chi can enhance flexibility, balance, and relaxation, which may aid in stress management and overall well-being.

4. **Low-impact activities:** For individuals with certain diabetes-related complications or joint issues, low-impact exercises like water aerobics or using an elliptical machine can be gentler on the body while still providing health benefits.

5. **Interval training:** Alternating between periods of high-intensity exercise and lower-intensity recovery periods can be an effective way to improve cardiovascular fitness and glucose control.

6. **Daily activities:** Even everyday activities like gardening, cleaning, or taking the stairs can

contribute to staying active and managing blood sugar levels.

Remember to start any exercise program gradually and listen to your body. Monitor your blood sugar levels before, during, and after exercise, and be prepared to adjust your diabetes management plan as needed. Always carry a source of fast-acting glucose, like glucose tablets or juice, in case of low blood sugar during or after physical activity.

Again, I can't emphasize enough the importance of consulting with a healthcare professional before starting any exercise regimen to ensure it is safe and suitable for your specific condition. They can provide personalized advice and help you create a plan that works best for you.

What exercise is best for a person that has had a knee replacement?

For individuals who have undergone knee replacement surgery, it is essential to engage in exercises that promote strength, flexibility, and mobility while being mindful of protecting the new knee joint. Exercise plays a crucial role in the rehabilitation process after knee replacement surgery, helping to regain function, reduce pain, and improve overall quality of life. However, it's important to consult with your orthopedic surgeon or physical therapist before starting any exercise program to ensure it is safe and appropriate for your specific condition and recovery stage. They can provide personalized guidance and recommendations based on your individual needs and progress. That being said, here are some exercises commonly recommended for people who have had knee replacement surgery:

1. **Range of motion exercises:** Gentle knee movements like bending and straightening the knee joint can help improve flexibility and prevent stiffness. Ankle pumps, heel slides, and knee flexion exercises are commonly prescribed in the early stages of recovery.

2. **Strengthening exercises:** Strengthening the muscles around the knee joint can provide support and stability. Initially, exercises may focus on the quadriceps (front thigh muscles) and progress to include the hamstrings and calf muscles. Leg lifts, seated leg extensions, and partial squats are examples of strengthening exercises.

3. **Stationary biking:** Cycling on a stationary bike is a low-impact exercise that can help improve knee joint mobility and strength without putting excessive stress on the joint. Start with a short duration and low resistance and gradually increase as tolerated.

4. **Water exercises:** Aquatic exercises, such as water walking or swimming, can be gentle on the knee joint while providing resistance to build strength and range of motion.

5. **Heel and calf raises:** These exercises can help strengthen the calf muscles and improve ankle flexibility.

6. **Leg press machine:** Once your surgeon or physical therapist approves, using a leg press machine with proper form can help build quadriceps strength.

7. **Seated or lying hamstring curls:** These exercises target the hamstring muscles, which are important for knee stability.

8. **Balance and stability exercises:** Improving balance can reduce the risk of falls and promote confidence in daily activities. Balance exercises may include standing on one leg, using a balance board, or practicing yoga.

Remember to progress gradually and avoid high-impact activities or exercises that put excessive strain on the knee joint, such as running or jumping, especially in the early stages of recovery. Listen to your body and stop any exercise that causes pain or discomfort.

Additionally, always follow the guidance and recommendations provided by your healthcare professionals regarding your specific post-surgery rehabilitation plan. They can monitor your progress and make adjustments as needed to ensure a safe and successful recovery.

What exercise is best for a person that has had hip replacement surgery ?

Before engaging in any exercise routine after hip replacement surgery, it's crucial to consult with your doctor or physical therapist to ensure it's safe and suitable for your specific condition. The best exercises for someone who has had a hip replacement surgery are those that help improve strength, flexibility, and overall function while minimizing the risk of injury. Here are some recommended exercises:

1. **Walking:** Walking is a low-impact activity that helps improve cardiovascular fitness and overall mobility. Start with short distances and gradually increase as you gain strength and confidence.

2. **Stationary biking:** Riding a stationary bike is gentle on the hips and provides an excellent way to improve strength and range of motion in the joint.

3. **Swimming:** Swimming and water aerobics are great options as they put minimal stress on the hip joint while providing a full-body workout.

4. **Leg raises:** Perform seated or lying leg raises to strengthen the muscles around the hip joint, such as the quadriceps and hip abductors.

5. **Bridges:** Lie on your back with your knees bent and feet flat on the floor. Lift your hips off the ground, engaging your glutes and core. Lower back down and repeat.

6. **Ankle pumps and circles:** These simple exercises can be done while lying down to improve blood circulation and maintain ankle mobility.

7. **Step-ups:** Using a low step or sturdy box, step up with the operated leg and then lower back down. This exercise helps build strength in the hip and leg muscles.

8. **Gentle stretches:** Perform gentle hip stretches to maintain flexibility and reduce stiffness in the joint.

What is the best exercise for a person that has had a liver transplant?

It is essential for someone who has had a liver transplant to engage in regular physical activity, as it can have numerous benefits, including improving overall health, boosting immune function, maintaining a healthy weight, and enhancing cardiovascular fitness. However, it is crucial to consult with the medical team and healthcare provider who oversaw the liver transplant to get personalized recommendations and ensure that exercise is safe and appropriate for the individual's specific condition and recovery stage. They can provide tailored advice based on the person's medical history, current health status, and any potential restrictions or limitations.

In general, the best exercise for someone who has had a liver transplant would be low-impact activities that gradually increase in intensity and duration over time. Some recommended exercises may include:

1. **Walking:** It is a low-impact activity that can be easily adjusted to the individual's fitness level and can help improve cardiovascular health and endurance.

2. **Swimming:** This is a great option as it is gentle on the joints and provides a full-body workout.

3. **Cycling:** Stationary or outdoor cycling can be suitable for improving cardiovascular fitness without putting excessive stress on the liver.

4. **Stretching and flexibility exercises:** These can help maintain joint mobility and prevent muscle tightness.

5. **Light resistance training:** Under professional supervision, gentle strength exercises can help rebuild muscle strength and improve overall fitness.

6. **Breathing exercises:** Breathing exercises can aid in relaxation and stress reduction, which is beneficial for overall well-being.

Remember, it is vital to start slowly and gradually progress the intensity and duration of the exercises. The medical team should be involved in designing an exercise program that aligns with the individual's health needs and capabilities. Additionally, any signs of discomfort, pain, or unusual symptoms during exercise should be reported to the healthcare provider promptly.

As always, it's essential to follow medical advice and attend regular follow-up appointments to ensure a safe and successful recovery after a liver transplant.

What is the absolute best way to lose weight ?

The absolute best way to lose weight can vary from person to person, as individual factors such as metabolism, body composition, lifestyle, and medical conditions play a significant role in weight loss. However, some general principles can guide most people on their weight loss journey:

1. **Balanced and Healthy Diet:** Focus on a well-balanced diet that includes a variety of nutrient-rich foods, such as fruits, vegetables, lean proteins, whole grains, and healthy fats. Avoid or limit sugary, processed, and high-calorie foods.

2. **Portion Control:** Watch your portion sizes to avoid overeating. Even healthy foods can contribute to weight gain if consumed in excessive amounts.

3. **Regular Exercise:** Engage in regular physical activity that you enjoy, such as walking, running, swimming, cycling, or strength training. Aim for at least 150 minutes of moderate-intensity aerobic exercise per week, combined with muscle-strengthening activities on two or more days a week.

4. **Stay Hydrated:** Drink plenty of water throughout the day, as it can help control appetite and support overall health.

5. **Adequate Sleep:** Ensure you get enough quality sleep each night. Poor sleep patterns can disrupt hormonal balances and lead to weight gain.

6. **Mindful Eating:** Pay attention to your hunger and fullness cues, and avoid emotional eating or eating out of boredom.

7. **Seek Professional Guidance:** If you have specific health concerns or medical conditions, consult with a healthcare professional or registered dietitian to create a personalized weight loss plan.

8. **Patience and Consistency:** Sustainable weight loss takes time and effort. Avoid crash diets or extreme approaches, as they can be harmful in the long run. Focus on creating healthy habits that you can maintain over time.

9. **Accountability and Support:** Consider joining a weight loss group or seeking support from friends, family, or a weight loss community to help you stay motivated and accountable.

Remember, weight loss is not just about a short-term goal but also about making positive lifestyle changes that you can maintain for the long term. Always prioritize your overall health and well-being while pursuing weight loss goals.

How much protein per pound does a person need each day

To calculate the recommended daily protein intake in grams per pound of body weight, you can use the following guidelines:

1. Sedentary Adults or Minimal Physical Activity: 0.36 grams of protein per pound of body weight per day.

2. Moderately Active Adults or Regular Exercise: 0.54 to 0.77 grams of protein per pound of body weight per day.

3. Very Active Individuals or Athletes: 0.63 to 1 gram of protein per pound of body weight per day.

For example, for a sedentary adult weighing 150 pounds, the protein intake would be around 54 grams per day (150 lbs x 0.36 g/lb). For a moderately active adult, the protein intake may range from 81 to 116 grams per day (150 lbs x 0.54 to 0.77 g/lb). And for a highly active individual, it may range from 95 to 150 grams per day (150 lbs x 0.63 to 1 g/lb).

These recommendations are approximate and meant to provide a general range of protein intake based on activity levels. As always, individual protein needs can vary, and it's best to consider other factors like age, gender, muscle mass, and specific health goals when determining your ideal protein intake.

For personalized dietary advice, it's advisable to consult with a registered dietitian or healthcare professional who can assess your unique needs and develop a tailored nutrition plan.

How much extra protein does a person need to build muscle?

When aiming to build muscle, individuals typically require more protein than those with maintenance or weight loss goals. Protein is essential for muscle repair and growth, and consuming an adequate amount can support the muscle-building process.

The amount of extra protein needed to build muscle can vary based on factors such as age, gender, current muscle mass, training intensity, and overall caloric intake. However, a common guideline used by many fitness experts and organizations is to aim for a protein intake of around 1.2 to 2.2 grams per kilogram of body weight per day for those engaged in resistance training or other forms of intense exercise to build muscle.

To calculate the recommended protein intake in grams per pound of body weight, you can use the following guideline:

1.2 to 2.2 grams of protein per kilogram of body weight per day.

For example, for a person weighing 150 pounds (approximately 68 kg) and engaged in resistance training to build muscle, the protein intake would range from approximately 82 to 150 grams per day (68 kg x 1.2 to 2.2 g/kg).

It's important to note that while protein is crucial for muscle building, other factors such as overall caloric intake, macronutrient distribution, training intensity, and recovery play significant roles in the muscle-building process. A balanced diet that includes enough calories from carbohydrates and fats, along with adequate protein, is essential for optimal muscle growth.

Again, individual protein needs may vary, and for personalized advice, it's recommended to consult with a registered dietitian or a healthcare professional who can assess your specific goals, training routine, and nutritional needs to develop an appropriate plan for muscle building.

How long does it take to build new muscle?

The time it takes to build new muscle, also known as muscle hypertrophy, can vary depending on several factors, including individual genetics, training intensity, frequency, nutrition, and recovery. There is no one-size-fits-all answer to this question, but generally, you can expect to see noticeable muscle growth within a few weeks to a few months of consistent and effective training.

Here are some general guidelines for muscle growth:

1. **Initial Strength Gain:** In the early stages of resistance training, especially if you are new to strength training, you may experience what is often called "neuromuscular adaptation." During this period, your body becomes more efficient at recruiting existing muscle fibers, leading to an increase in

strength without significant muscle size gains. This phase can occur within the first few weeks of training.

2. **Visible Muscle Growth:** Noticeable muscle growth typically starts becoming apparent within 4 to 8 weeks of consistent training. This is when muscle fibers are subjected to enough stress to trigger the muscle repair and growth process.

3. **Significant Muscle Growth:** For most people, significant muscle hypertrophy occurs within 3 to 6 months of consistent and progressive resistance training. This time frame can vary, and some individuals might experience faster progress, while others might take longer.

4. **Long-term Progress:** Building muscle is an ongoing process. Continued training, proper nutrition, and adequate recovery will contribute to continuous muscle gains over months and years of consistent effort.

Keep in mind that everyone's body responds differently to training, and genetics play a significant role in determining how quickly you can build muscle. Additionally, factors like age, hormone levels, and overall health can also influence muscle growth.

Consistency, progressive overload (gradually increasing the resistance or intensity of your workouts), and a balanced diet with enough protein are essential elements for muscle growth. Remember that building muscle is a gradual process that requires patience and dedication.

What is the best way to get rid of stubborn belly fat?

Getting rid of stubborn belly fat requires a combination of healthy lifestyle choices, including diet, exercise, and stress management. Here are some effective strategies to help you achieve your goal:

1. **Balanced Diet:** Focus on a balanced and nutritious diet. Reduce your calorie intake and aim to consume more whole foods like fruits, vegetables, lean proteins, and whole grains. Avoid sugary drinks and processed foods.

2. **Portion Control:** Be mindful of your portion sizes to prevent overeating. Even healthy foods can contribute to weight gain if consumed in large quantities.

3. **Hydration:** Drink plenty of water throughout the day. Sometimes, thirst can be mistaken for hunger, leading to unnecessary snacking.

4. **Regular Exercise:** Incorporate both cardiovascular exercises (such as running, swimming, or cycling) and strength training (like weightlifting or bodyweight exercises) into your routine. Regular exercise can help burn calories and build muscle, which can increase your metabolism.

5. **HIIT (High-Intensity Interval Training):** Consider including high-intensity interval training in your exercise routine. This type of workout alternates between short bursts of intense activity and brief rest periods, helping to burn more calories in less time.

6. **Core Exercises:** Include exercises that specifically target your abdominal muscles, such as crunches, planks, and leg raises. While spot reduction is not effective, strengthening your core can help improve muscle tone and posture.

7. **Reduce Stress:** Chronic stress can lead to weight gain, including belly fat. Practice stress-reduction techniques like meditation, yoga, deep breathing, or spending time doing activities you enjoy.

8. **Adequate Sleep:** Make sure to get enough quality sleep each night. Lack of sleep can disrupt your hormones and increase your appetite, leading to weight gain.

9. **Avoid Crash Diets:** Avoid extreme or crash diets, as they are unsustainable and can lead to muscle loss, nutrient deficiencies, and a rebound effect once you stop the diet.

10. **Be Patient and Consistent:** Losing belly fat takes time, and everyone's body responds differently. Stay committed to your healthy lifestyle changes, and remember that slow, steady progress is more sustainable in the long run.

It's essential to consult with a healthcare professional or a registered dietitian before making significant changes to your diet or exercise routine, especially if you have any underlying health conditions or concerns. They can provide personalized guidance and support to help you reach your goals safely and effectively.

What are the best exercises for a person with a heart defribilator

If you have a heart defibrillator (also known as an implantable cardioverter-defibrillator or ICD), it's crucial to prioritize safety and avoid certain exercises that may interfere with the device's proper functioning or put undue stress on your heart. Always consult with your healthcare provider before starting any exercise program, as they can provide personalized recommendations based on your specific medical condition and the type of ICD you have. Generally, exercises that are low-impact and avoid sudden, intense movements are considered safer for individuals with an ICD. Here are some exercises that may be suitable:

1. **Walking:** Walking is a low-impact and accessible exercise that provides cardiovascular benefits without putting excessive strain on your heart. Aim for brisk walks, especially if your doctor approves.

2. **Swimming:** Swimming is an excellent full-body workout that is gentle on your joints and heart. Make sure to avoid swimming in excessively cold or hot water, as extreme temperatures can affect your ICD.

3. **Cycling:** Riding a stationary bike or cycling outdoors at a moderate pace can be a safe cardiovascular exercise.

4. **Yoga:** Gentle yoga classes that focus on breathing, stretching, and relaxation can be beneficial for overall well-being and stress management.

5. **Tai Chi:** Tai Chi is a slow, low-impact exercise that promotes balance, flexibility, and relaxation.

6. **Resistance Training:** Light resistance exercises using bands or light weights can help maintain muscle tone and strength. Avoid heavy lifting or exercises that involve straining.

7. **Pilates:** Pilates can be modified to suit different fitness levels and focuses on core strength, flexibility, and controlled movements.

8. **Elliptical Trainer:** Using an elliptical machine can provide a low-impact cardiovascular workout without putting excessive stress on your heart.

Remember to start slowly and gradually increase the intensity and duration of your exercises as you become more comfortable and confident. Pay attention to any signs of discomfort, chest pain, palpitations, or shortness of breath, and stop exercising immediately if you experience any concerning symptoms.

Always wear appropriate medical identification, inform your exercise instructors about your condition, and follow your doctor's guidance on exercise limitations and safety precautions. Regular check-ups with your healthcare provider are essential to monitor the function of your ICD and ensure your exercise plan remains suitable for your specific health needs.

What are good exercises for a person who has had a double mastectomy?

It's important to note that exercise recommendations can vary based on individual health conditions, medical history, and personal preferences. If someone has undergone a double mastectomy, they should always consult with their healthcare provider before beginning any exercise program. That being said, here are some general guidelines and potential exercises that might be beneficial for individuals who have had a double mastectomy:

1. **Range of Motion Exercises:** Gentle range of motion exercises can help maintain flexibility and prevent stiffness in the shoulder and chest area. These exercises might include shoulder circles, arm swings, and wall slides.

2. **Deep Breathing Exercises:** Deep breathing exercises can help improve lung capacity and promote relaxation. Focus on slow, controlled breathing to expand the chest and promote healing.

3. **Stretching:** Gentle stretching can help improve flexibility and alleviate tension in the chest, shoulder, and upper back muscles. Stretching exercises should be done cautiously and with proper guidance.

4. **Resistance Training:** Light resistance exercises can help strengthen the muscles around the chest, shoulders, and back. Start with very light weights or resistance bands, and gradually increase intensity as tolerated. Examples include seated rows, chest presses (if approved by a healthcare professional), and bicep curls.

5. **Aerobic Exercises:** Low-impact aerobic exercises like walking, stationary cycling, and swimming (once healed and cleared by a healthcare professional) can help improve cardiovascular fitness and overall well-being.

6. **Posture Improvement:** Focus on exercises that help improve posture, as this can contribute to better alignment and reduced strain on the chest and shoulder area. Exercises that target the upper back and core can be beneficial.

7. **Yoga or Pilates:** Gentle yoga or Pilates classes specifically designed for post-surgery patients can help improve flexibility, strength, and body awareness. Look for classes that are led by instructors who have experience working with individuals who have undergone mastectomies.

8. **Walking:** Walking is a low-impact exercise that promotes circulation, improves mood, and supports overall health. Start with short walks and gradually increase the duration and intensity as you feel comfortable.

Remember to prioritize safety and listen to your body. If any exercise causes discomfort or pain, stop immediately and consult your healthcare provider. Always follow your doctor's recommendations and guidelines for exercise after a double mastectomy. They can provide personalized advice based on your specific situation and recovery progress.

How long does it take to lower blood pressure through exercise?

The time it takes to lower blood pressure through exercise can vary widely depending on several factors, including your current fitness level, the type and intensity of exercise, how consistently you engage in physical activity, and your overall health. Here are some general guidelines to keep in mind:

1. **Short-Term Effects:** Engaging in a single bout of aerobic exercise, such as brisk walking, jogging, or cycling, can lead to temporary reductions in blood pressure that last for several hours after the exercise session. This short-term effect is known as post-exercise hypotension.

2. **Long-Term Effects:** To achieve sustained and long-term reductions in blood pressure, it's recommended to engage in regular physical activity over an extended period. Consistency is key. Over time, regular exercise can lead to improvements in cardiovascular health, including lower resting blood pressure.

3. **Timeline:** Some individuals may start to notice improvements in their blood pressure within a few weeks to a few months of consistently engaging in a well-rounded exercise routine. However, significant and lasting changes may take several months to a year or more of regular exercise.

4. **Individual Variation:** Everyone responds differently to exercise. Some individuals may experience faster reductions in blood pressure due to genetic factors, existing fitness levels, and overall health.

5. **Combining with Other Lifestyle Changes:** Keep in mind that exercise is most effective when combined with other healthy lifestyle changes, such as a balanced diet, stress management, and maintaining a healthy weight. These factors work together to support better blood pressure control.

6. **Consult a Healthcare Provider:** It's essential to consult with your healthcare provider before starting an exercise program, especially if you have existing health conditions, including high blood pressure. They can provide personalized recommendations based on your individual health needs.

Remember that improving cardiovascular health is a gradual process, and consistency is key. It's important to set realistic expectations and focus on making sustainable lifestyle changes that contribute to better overall health in the long run. If you have high blood pressure or are at risk for cardiovascular issues, working with healthcare professionals can help you monitor your progress and make informed decisions about your exercise and health goals.

What is the best way to quit smoking?

Quitting smoking is a challenging but highly rewarding endeavor that can significantly improve your health and well-being. Here are some effective strategies to help you quit smoking:

1. **Commit to Quit:** Make a firm decision to quit smoking and set a quit date. Choose a date within the next few weeks to give yourself time to prepare mentally and emotionally.

2. **Seek Support:**

    - **Healthcare Provider:** Consult your healthcare provider for guidance and support. They can provide personalized advice, prescribe medications, and monitor your progress.

    - **Counseling:** Consider individual or group counseling, behavioral therapy, or support groups to help you address the psychological and emotional aspects of quitting.

3. **Nicotine Replacement Therapy (NRT):** NRT products, such as nicotine gum, patches, lozenges, nasal spray, or inhalers, can help manage withdrawal symptoms by providing controlled doses of nicotine. These can increase your chances of quitting successfully.

4. **Prescription Medications:** Talk to your doctor about prescription medications that can help reduce nicotine cravings and withdrawal symptoms. Examples include varenicline (Chantix) and bupropion (Zyban).

5. **Identify Triggers:** Recognize situations, emotions, or activities that trigger your smoking habit. Develop strategies to cope with these triggers, such as finding healthier alternatives or practicing relaxation techniques.

6. **Change Habits:** Replace smoking with healthier habits. Engage in physical activities, hobbies, or activities that keep your mind and hands busy.

7. **Avoid Smoking Environments:** Stay away from places or situations that encourage smoking, especially during the initial stages of quitting.

8. **Stay Hydrated:** Drink plenty of water to help flush nicotine and toxins from your body.

9. **Practice Stress Management:** Learn and use stress-reduction techniques such as deep breathing, meditation, yoga, or progressive muscle relaxation.

10. **Reward Yourself:** Celebrate milestones, whether they're small or significant, to recognize your progress and commitment.

11. **Prepare for Withdrawal:** Understand that withdrawal symptoms like irritability, cravings, and

mood swings are temporary. They will lessen over time.

12. **Visualize Success:** Imagine yourself as a non-smoker and focus on the health benefits and positive changes that come with quitting.

13. **Learn from Relapses:** If you slip up and smoke, don't get discouraged. It's a common part of the quitting process. Analyze what triggered the relapse and use it as an opportunity to strengthen your commitment.

14. **Stay Persistent:** Quitting smoking may take multiple attempts. Don't give up even if you face challenges along the way.

15. **Supportive Environment:** Inform your family and friends about your decision to quit. Ask for their support and encouragement.

Remember, quitting smoking is a journey that requires patience, determination, and resilience. It's a positive step toward improving your health and quality of life. If you find it challenging, don't hesitate to seek professional help and utilize the available resources to increase your chances of success.

Is there such a thing as detoxifiy your body?

The concept of "detoxifying" the body is often discussed in the context of various health practices, diets, and products. However, it's important to approach this concept with a critical and science-based perspective.

1. **Detoxification by Organs:** The human body has built-in mechanisms for detoxification. Organs like the liver, kidneys, and lungs are responsible for filtering and eliminating toxins from the body. These organs work continuously to process waste products and maintain internal balance.

2. **Misleading Claims:** Many commercial detox products or diets claim to cleanse the body of accumulated toxins, improve energy levels, and promote overall health. However, the scientific evidence supporting the effectiveness of these claims is often limited or lacking.

3. **Unproven Methods:** Some detox methods involve fasting, extreme calorie restriction, consuming specific juices or herbal supplements, or undergoing colon cleansing procedures. These methods can be potentially harmful, disrupt normal bodily functions, and lack scientific validation.

4. **Weight Loss vs. Detoxification:** Some people may perceive weight loss as a sign of successful detoxification, but weight loss often occurs due to reduced calorie intake rather than the elimination of toxins.

5. **Balanced Nutrition:** Instead of extreme detox diets, focus on a balanced and nutritious diet that supports the body's natural detoxification processes. Consuming a variety of whole foods, plenty of fruits and vegetables, lean proteins, and adequate hydration can support overall health.

6. **Healthy Lifestyle Choices:** Adopting healthy lifestyle habits, including regular exercise, adequate sleep, stress management, and avoiding excessive alcohol and processed foods, can contribute to optimal organ function and overall well-being.

7. **Consulting Professionals:** If you're concerned about specific toxins or heavy metals in your body, it's best to consult a healthcare provider. They can assess your individual situation and recommend appropriate testing and interventions if necessary.

In summary, while there is no one-size-fits-all "detox" solution, the body's natural detoxification systems function efficiently when supported by a healthy lifestyle. Rather than relying on extreme diets or products, focus on making sustainable choices that promote your overall health and well-being. If you have concerns about toxins or health issues, seek guidance from qualified healthcare professionals.

Is there such a thing a liver detox

The term "liver detox" is often used in alternative medicine and wellness circles to refer to various practices and products that are claimed to help the liver remove toxins from the body and improve its function. However, the concept of a "liver detox" is not fully supported by mainstream medical science.

The liver is a vital organ responsible for metabolizing nutrients, filtering blood, and eliminating waste products and toxins from the body. It performs these functions naturally and continuously without the need for specific detoxification processes or interventions. The liver processes toxins and waste products through complex enzymatic reactions and then excretes them through bile and urine.

Many of the claims made about liver detoxification methods, such as detox diets, fasting, juice cleanses, herbal supplements, and special detoxifying products, lack substantial scientific evidence. While some of these practices might lead to short-term changes in how you feel or even slight changes in liver enzyme levels, there is little evidence to suggest that they significantly enhance the liver's natural detoxification abilities.

It's 'mportant to note that extreme detoxification practices or diets could potentially do more harm than good. For instance, crash diets or restrictive diets can deprive the body of essential nutrients and lead to adverse health effects.

If you're concerned about your liver health or overall well-being, it's always best to consult with a qualified medical professional. They can provide personalized advice based on your medical history and current health status. If you're interested in supporting your liver health, maintaining a balanced diet, staying hydrated, getting regular exercise, and avoiding excessive alcohol consumption are generally recommended practices.

What Are The Top Five Foundational Supplements You Should Consider Taking If You Are Near Fifty or Older?

In this fast-paced world our bodies need a little extra help to stay functioning at our best. That's where vitamins come in. They give our body that extra boost to help you stay fit and feeling and looking younger.

First lest start with the disclaimer. This article is not intended to disburse medical advice. Everything is not for everybody. For example, while Vitamin K is not one of the top five, if you are on warfarin or other blood thinners you should not be taking vitamin K supplements. Consult your healthcare professional for medical advice.

These recommendations are based upon exhaustive research of scientific literature, peer reviewed articles, interviews with doctors researchers and professionals in the health supplement industry.

The Top Five Are:

1. Vitamin D3

2. Vitamin B3 (Niacinamide)
3. Curcumin
4. Hydrolyzed Collagen
5. Co Q 10

1. Vitamin D works with calcium to support your bones and has also been shown to help strengthen muscles. It may play a role in regulating mood and protecting from viruses bacteria and respiratory tract infections. Studies have also shown that vitamin D helps fight inflammation and having adequate levels of Vitamin D may help prevent heart disease, stroke, high blood pressure and heart attacks.

2. Vitamin B3 also known as niacin plays a role in regulating good cholesterol by helping the body use proteins fats and converting food into energy. It helps maintain a healthy nervous system and is good for the skin and hair.

3. Curcumin, a natural STAT 3 inhibitor has been researched and may play a role in the prevention of certain cancers, Researchers are also looking into its role in delaying Alzheimer's, treating arthritis, and controlling diabetes

4. Hydrolyzed Collagen is one of the most researched supplements for shin health, skin elasticity and smoothing out wrinkles. Growing research has found that collagen helps to manage chronic joint pain, skeletal muscular and is a great nutrient for the lining of the gut. Hydrolyzed Collagen has been

broken down through the process of hydrolysis to make the is easier to be absorbed.

5. Co Q 10 decreases as we age. Co Q 10 has been shown to help improve the health of the heart while regulating blood sugar. It is said to also support prevention of periodontal disease, support brain and lung health and improve exercise performance.

You Can Find These Foundational Supplements In The Your Phenomenal Life Store:
https://yourphenomenallife.net/store

Can exercise help with erectile dysfunction?

Yes, exercise can potentially help with erectile dysfunction (ED) to some extent. Erectile dysfunction is the inability to achieve or maintain an erection sufficient for sexual activity. It can have various causes, including physical, psychological, and lifestyle factors. Regular exercise can address some of these factors and contribute to improved sexual health. Here's how exercise can be beneficial:

1. **Cardiovascular Health:** Many cases of ED are linked to poor blood circulation, which can result from underlying cardiovascular issues. Regular cardiovascular exercise, such as brisk walking, running, cycling, or swimming, can improve blood flow, strengthen the heart, and enhance overall cardiovascular health. Better blood flow can positively impact the ability to achieve and maintain an erection.

2. **Weight Management:** Obesity is a risk factor for both cardiovascular problems and ED. Engaging in regular exercise can help you maintain a healthy weight or lose excess weight, which in turn can improve hormonal balance and overall sexual health.

3. **Hormonal Balance:** Exercise, especially resistance training like weightlifting, can boost testosterone levels. Testosterone is a hormone that plays a role in sexual function and libido. Maintaining healthy testosterone levels can have a positive impact on sexual health.

4. **Stress Reduction:** Psychological factors, such as stress and anxiety, can contribute to ED. Exercise is known to reduce stress and trigger the release of endorphins, which are "feel-good" hormones that can improve mood and alleviate anxiety.

5. **Diabetes Management:** Diabetes is a common cause of ED. Regular exercise can help manage blood sugar levels and improve insulin sensitivity, which can in turn reduce the risk of diabetes-related ED.

6. **Pelvic Floor Muscles:** Certain exercises, such as Kegel exercises, can strengthen the pelvic floor muscles, which play a role in erectile function and ejaculation control.

It's important to note that while exercise can offer benefits for sexual health, it might not be a sole solution for everyone with ED. If you're experiencing persistent or severe erectile dysfunction, it's recommended to consult a healthcare professional. They can help identify the underlying causes of your condition and recommend appropriate treatments or interventions, which might include lifestyle changes, medications, or other therapies.

What is the best way to keep the brain fit as we age?

Keeping the brain fit as you age involves a combination of lifestyle choices, activities, and habits that promote cognitive health. Here are some effective strategies to consider:

1. **Stay Physically Active:** Regular physical exercise has been linked to improved cognitive function and a reduced risk of cognitive decline. Activities like brisk walking, jogging, swimming, and dancing can help improve blood flow to the brain and promote the growth of new neurons.

2. **Maintain a Healthy Diet:** A diet rich in fruits, vegetables, whole grains, lean proteins, and healthy fats can provide essential nutrients that support brain health. Omega-3 fatty acids, antioxidants, and vitamins like B-complex vitamins are particularly beneficial.

3. **Stay Mentally Active:** Engage in activities that challenge your brain regularly. This could include puzzles, crosswords, sudoku, reading, learning a new instrument, or a new language. Lifelong learning keeps the brain engaged and can help build cognitive reserve.

4. **Socialize:** Regular social interactions are associated with better cognitive health. Engaging in conversations, joining clubs or social groups, and spending time with friends and family can help keep your mind active and reduce the risk of isolation-related cognitive decline.

5. **Get Adequate Sleep:** Sleep is essential for cognitive function and memory consolidation. Aim for 7-9 hours of quality sleep each night. Establish a regular sleep schedule and create a comfortable sleep environment.

6. **Manage Stress:** Chronic stress can have a negative impact on brain health. Practice stress-reduction techniques such as meditation, mindfulness, deep breathing, yoga, or spending time in nature.

7. **Stay Hydrated:** Dehydration can affect cognitive function. Make sure to drink enough water throughout the day to maintain proper hydration.

8. **Challenge Your Brain:** Engage in activities that require problem-solving, critical thinking, and creativity. Learning new skills, taking up hobbies, and tackling complex tasks can stimulate brain growth.

9. **Limit Alcohol and Avoid Smoking:** Excessive alcohol consumption and smoking have been linked to cognitive decline. If you choose to consume alcohol, do so in moderation, and consider quitting smoking.

10. **Manage Chronic Conditions:** Conditions like diabetes, hypertension, and heart disease can impact brain health. Work with your healthcare provider to manage these conditions effectively.

11. **Stay Curious and Open-Minded:** Maintain a curious attitude toward life and stay open to new experiences. Novelty and curiosity stimulate brain activity and encourage learning.

12. **Stay Positive:** A positive outlook and emotional well-being contribute to cognitive health. Cultivate gratitude, practice mindfulness, and engage in activities that bring you joy.

Remember that brain health is a lifelong endeavor. It's never too late to start adopting these practices, even if you're already in your senior years. It's also important to consult with a healthcare professional if you have specific concerns about cognitive health or any underlying medical conditions.

How do you know if you are out of shape?

Being "out of shape" generally refers to a lower level of physical fitness or conditioning. It's important to note that fitness levels can vary widely from person to person, and being out of shape doesn't necessarily mean you're unhealthy. However, if you're wondering whether you're out of shape, here are some signs to consider:

1. **Shortness of Breath:** If you find yourself easily becoming short of breath after mild physical activities like climbing stairs or walking short

distances, it could be an indication that your cardiovascular fitness is not optimal.

2. **Fatigue:** Feeling tired or fatigued even after light physical exertion can be a sign of decreased fitness levels.

3. **Low Stamina:** If you're unable to engage in physical activities for an extended period without feeling exhausted, it might suggest that your endurance is lower than desired.

4. **Muscle Weakness:** Struggling to perform everyday tasks that require strength, like lifting groceries or carrying items, might indicate reduced muscle strength.

5. **Inflexibility:** If you have limited flexibility and find it challenging to perform basic stretches or movements, it could indicate that your body's range of motion is compromised.

6. **Poor Balance:** Difficulty maintaining balance or feeling unsteady during simple activities can be an indicator of reduced physical fitness.

7. **Weight Gain:** A sudden or gradual increase in body weight without changes in diet could be a sign that your activity level has decreased, leading to a decrease in overall fitness.

8. **Elevated Resting Heart Rate:** If your resting heart rate is consistently higher than usual, it might

suggest that your cardiovascular system is not as efficient as it could be.

9. **Difficulty Engaging in Physical Activities:** Struggling to participate in sports or recreational activities that you used to enjoy might indicate a decline in your physical fitness level.

10. **Health Conditions:** If you have health conditions such as high blood pressure, diabetes, or high cholesterol, they could be related to being out of shape.

It's important to remember that physical fitness is a gradual process that can be improved with consistent effort and appropriate exercise. If you're concerned about your fitness level, consider starting a regular exercise routine that includes cardiovascular workouts, strength training, and flexibility exercises. Consult with a healthcare professional before making significant changes to your exercise regimen, especially if you have any underlying health conditions. A healthcare provider or fitness professional can help you develop a safe and effective fitness plan tailored to your individual needs and goals.

What is the best way to maintain a healthy gut?

Maintaining a healthy gut is important for overall well-being, as the gut plays a crucial role in digestion, nutrient absorption, immune function, and even mental health. Here are some strategies to help you maintain a healthy gut:

1. **Eat a Diverse Diet:** Consume a wide variety of whole, nutrient-rich foods. Fiber-rich foods like fruits, vegetables, whole grains, legumes, and nuts can promote the growth of beneficial gut bacteria.

2. **Include Fermented Foods:** Fermented foods like yogurt, kefir, sauerkraut, kimchi, kombucha, and miso contain probiotics (beneficial bacteria) that can contribute to a healthy gut microbiome.

3. **Probiotic Supplements:** Consider taking probiotic supplements, especially if you have specific digestive issues or after a course of antibiotics. Consult with a healthcare professional before starting any supplements.

4. **Prebiotic Foods:** Prebiotics are non-digestible fibers that feed beneficial gut bacteria. Foods like garlic, onions, leeks, asparagus, and bananas are good sources of prebiotics.

5. **Stay Hydrated:** Drinking plenty of water supports healthy digestion and maintains the mucosal lining of the intestines.

6. **Limit Processed Foods:** Highly processed and sugary foods can negatively impact gut health by promoting the growth of harmful bacteria. Opt for whole foods as much as possible.

7. **Manage Stress:** Chronic stress can affect gut health. Practice stress-reduction techniques like meditation, deep breathing, yoga, or spending time in nature.

8. **Get Regular Exercise:** Physical activity can positively influence gut health by promoting a balanced gut microbiome and improving overall digestion.

9. **Adequate Sleep:** Prioritize getting 7-9 hours of quality sleep each night, as sleep is essential for maintaining a healthy gut.

10. **Avoid Antibiotics Unnecessarily:** Antibiotics can disrupt the balance of gut bacteria. Use antibiotics only when prescribed by a healthcare professional and consider probiotics during and after the course, if recommended.

11. **Limit Antibacterial Products:** Excessive use of antibacterial soaps and cleansers can negatively impact the diversity of your gut microbiome.

12. **Avoid Overuse of Pain Relievers:** Nonsteroidal anti-inflammatory drugs (NSAIDs) can irritate the gut lining. If you need to use them, do so in moderation.

13. **Stay Hygienic:** Wash your hands regularly and follow good hygiene practices to prevent harmful bacteria from entering your body.

14. **Mindful Eating:** Chew your food thoroughly, eat slowly, and pay attention to hunger and fullness cues. This supports healthy digestion.

15. **Limit Artificial Sweeteners:** Some artificial sweeteners may disrupt the gut microbiota. Opt for natural sweeteners in moderation if needed.

Remember that everyone's gut microbiome is unique, so what works best for one person might not work the same way for another. If you have specific gut-related concerns or digestive issues, it's recommended to consult with a healthcare professional or a registered dietitian who can provide personalized advice based on your individual needs and health status.

What is that crackling sound I hear when I begin to exercise?

The crackling or popping sound that you might hear when you begin to exercise, especially during movements like squats, lunges, or other leg exercises, is often referred to as "crepitus." Crepitus is the noise produced when there's friction between surfaces within a joint or between soft tissues around the joint. It can occur in various parts of the body, including the knees, hips, shoulders, and even the spine.

There are a few potential explanations for the crackling sound during exercise:

1. **Gas Bubble Release:** One common cause of crepitus is the release of gas bubbles from the synovial fluid in the joints. Synovial fluid helps lubricate the joints and reduce friction. When you move your joints, such as during exercise, these gas bubbles can escape and create a popping or crackling sound.

2. **Tendon or Ligament Movement:** The sound might also be due to tendons or ligaments moving over bony prominences or other tissues. This movement can create a popping sensation or noise.

3. **Joint Alignment Changes:** During exercise, your joint alignment and movement patterns change. If the joint surfaces or tissues are not moving smoothly or are slightly misaligned, it can lead to crepitus.

4. **Muscle Contractions:** Sometimes, the sound could be related to muscle contractions causing movement or pressure changes around the joint.

In many cases, crepitus is harmless and doesn't cause pain or discomfort. However, if you experience pain, swelling, instability, or any other unusual symptoms along with the cracking sounds, it's important to consult a healthcare professional, such as a sports medicine doctor or physical therapist. They can assess your situation, determine the cause of the crepitus, and recommend any necessary interventions or modifications to your exercise routine.

It's worth noting that while crepitus is often harmless, persistent or painful cracking sounds could be a sign of an underlying issue that should be addressed by a medical professional. If you're concerned about the sounds you're experiencing, it's always a good idea to get expert advice to ensure your joint health and overall well-being.

How long does it usually take broken bones to heal?

The time it takes for a broken bone to heal can vary widely depending on several factors, including the type and location of the fracture, your age, overall health, and the treatment you receive. In general, bone healing can take several weeks to months. Here's a general overview of the healing timeline:

1. **Inflammation (Days 1-7):** When a bone breaks, the body responds with inflammation at the site of the fracture. Blood vessels dilate to bring in immune cells and healing factors. A blood clot forms, and a soft callus begins to develop around the fractured ends of the bone.

2. **Repair (Weeks 1-6):** The soft callus gradually transforms into a harder, woven bone structure. This process is called "callus formation." New blood vessels grow into the callus, providing nutrients for bone cell growth.

3. **Consolidation (Weeks 6-12):** The callus continues to strengthen and mineralize, forming a hard callus. During this phase, the bone starts to regain its structural integrity. Immature bone cells (osteoblasts) continue to replace the soft callus with more organized, mature bone tissue.

4. **Remodeling (Months 3-9+):** The newly formed bone undergoes a process of remodeling, where excess bone tissue is resorbed by cells called osteoclasts and replaced with compact bone. This process can take

several months and is influenced by your activity level and the mechanical stresses placed on the healing bone.

The overall healing time can be influenced by various factors:

- **Fracture Type:** Simple fractures (those with clean breaks) often heal faster than complex fractures (those with multiple pieces or involving joints).

- **Location:** Bones with better blood supply, like the forearm, may heal more quickly than bones with limited blood supply, like the femur.

- **Age:** Younger individuals tend to heal faster due to better cell activity and blood flow.

- **Health:** Conditions like diabetes or poor circulation can slow healing.

- **Treatment:** Immobilization with casts, splints, or even surgical fixation can impact healing time.

As a rough estimate:

- **Simple Fractures:** Can take around 6-8 weeks to heal in healthy adults.

- **Complex Fractures:** May require 10-16 weeks or more.

- **Long Bones (e.g., femur):** Can take several months to fully heal and remodel.

Remember that the healing process is not linear, and individual cases can vary. Always follow your healthcare provider's recommendations for treatment, activity restrictions, and follow-up appointments. They will monitor your progress and adjust your treatment plan as needed to ensure proper healing.

Why is oral hygiene important to overall fitness?

Oral hygiene is important not only for maintaining a healthy mouth but also for overall fitness and well-being. Here are several reasons why oral hygiene is closely connected to your overall health:

1. **Oral-Systemic Connection:** The health of your mouth is interconnected with the health of your entire body. Poor oral hygiene can contribute to various systemic health issues, including cardiovascular disease, diabetes, respiratory infections, and more.

2. **Inflammation and Immune Response:** Infections and inflammation in the mouth, such as gum disease (periodontitis), can trigger an immune response that affects other parts of the body. Chronic inflammation is associated with a range of health problems.

3. **Cardiovascular Health:** There's evidence of a link between gum disease and an increased risk of cardiovascular diseases like heart attacks and strokes. The bacteria from oral infections can enter

the bloodstream and contribute to inflammation in blood vessels.

4. **Diabetes Management:** Gum disease can make it harder to control blood sugar levels in people with diabetes, and diabetes itself can increase the risk of gum disease. Proper oral hygiene can help manage this interaction.

5. **Respiratory Health:** Bacteria from the mouth can be aspirated into the lungs, potentially leading to respiratory infections or exacerbating existing respiratory conditions.

6. **Nutrition and Eating Habits:** Dental issues can affect your ability to chew and enjoy a varied diet. Maintaining good oral health supports proper nutrition and overall health.

7. **Prevention of Infections:** Regular brushing and flossing help prevent the buildup of plaque, which can lead to cavities, gum disease, and infections that can impact overall health.

8. **Digestion:** Good oral health starts with proper chewing and digestion of food, which is essential for nutrient absorption and overall digestive health.

9. **Self-Confidence and Mental Well-Being:** Maintaining healthy teeth and gums can improve your self-esteem and mental well-being, contributing to overall fitness and quality of life.

10. **Sleep Quality:** Conditions like sleep apnea and teeth grinding (bruxism) can impact sleep quality and overall health. Some dental issues may contribute to these conditions.

To maintain good oral hygiene:

- Brush your teeth twice a day with fluoride toothpaste.

- Floss daily to clean between teeth and along the gumline.

- Use mouthwash if recommended by your dentist.

- Visit your dentist regularly for check-ups and cleanings.

- Limit sugary and acidic foods and drinks that can contribute to tooth decay.

- Quit smoking or using tobacco products, as they can harm oral health.

- Address any dental issues promptly to prevent complications.

By practicing good oral hygiene habits, you're not only promoting a healthy mouth but also contributing to your overall fitness and well-being. Regular dental care is an important part of your holistic health routine.

Can you have sex in your nineties?

Yes, it is possible for people in their nineties to engage in sexual activity, but there are several factors to consider. Sexual health is a normal and natural part of life, and age does not necessarily preclude sexual activity. However, there are a few things to keep in mind:

1. **Individual Health:** The ability to engage in sexual activity can be influenced by an individual's overall health and well-being. People in their nineties may have varying degrees of physical health, mobility, and energy levels.

2. **Partner's Health:** If you have a partner, their health and comfort levels are also important. Open and honest communication is key to understanding each other's needs and limitations.

3. **Communication:** It's important to communicate openly with your partner about your desires, expectations, and any concerns you may have. Discussing preferences, comfort levels, and any potential challenges can lead to a more satisfying and enjoyable experience.

4. **Physical Considerations:** As we age, certain physical changes may occur that can impact sexual activity, such as changes in hormone levels, vaginal dryness, and erectile function. These issues can often be addressed with the help of medical professionals.

5. **Emotional and Psychological Factors:** Emotional intimacy and a strong emotional connection with a partner can greatly enhance sexual experiences. Feeling safe, valued, and loved can contribute to a positive sexual experience.

6. **Safe Practices:** If engaging in sexual activity, it's important to consider safe practices to prevent sexually transmitted infections (STIs). Using protection, such as condoms, can help reduce the risk of STIs.

7. **Consulting Healthcare Professionals:** If you have specific health concerns or medical conditions, it's a good idea to consult with a healthcare provider to ensure that sexual activity is safe for you and your partner.

Ultimately, the decision to engage in sexual activity is a personal one that should be based on mutual consent, comfort, and respect for yourself and your partner. While physical limitations can arise with age, maintaining a healthy lifestyle, communicating openly with your partner, and seeking appropriate medical guidance can contribute to a positive and fulfilling sexual experience for those in their nineties and beyond.

How long does it take for muscles to grow when exercising?

The time it takes for muscles to grow (muscle hypertrophy) varies based on several factors, including your genetics, exercise routine, nutrition, rest, and overall consistency. Here's a general overview of what you can expect:

1. **Initial Strength Gains:** In the first few weeks of starting a new exercise routine, you might experience initial strength gains due to improved neuromuscular coordination and efficiency. This is not necessarily muscle hypertrophy but rather your body becoming more adept at using the existing muscle fibers.

2. **Visible Changes:** Visible muscle growth typically becomes noticeable after a few weeks to a few months of consistent training. This can vary widely based on individual factors. Some people may see changes sooner, while others might take longer.

3. **Adaptation and Progression:** As your muscles adapt to the stress of resistance training, you'll need to progressively increase the challenge to continue stimulating growth. This can be achieved by gradually increasing the weight, intensity, or volume of your workouts.

4. **Timeline:** Generally, significant muscle growth can take several months to a year of consistent and targeted resistance training. After about six months

of consistent training, you might see noticeable changes in your muscle size and definition.

5. **Plateaus:** It's common to experience periods of slower progress or plateaus in muscle growth. This is normal and can be overcome by adjusting your training routine, nutrition, and recovery strategies.

6. **Genetics:** Genetics play a role in how quickly and to what extent your muscles grow. Some individuals may naturally have an easier time building muscle, while others might progress more slowly.

7. **Nutrition:** Proper nutrition is essential for muscle growth. Consuming enough protein and overall calories to support your workouts and recovery is crucial.

8. **Recovery:** Muscles need time to recover and repair after intense workouts. Make sure to get adequate sleep and allow enough rest between training sessions to promote optimal muscle growth.

Remember that muscle growth is a gradual process, and consistency is key. It's important to have realistic expectations and avoid comparing your progress to others, as everyone's journey is unique. If you're new to resistance training, consider working with a fitness professional to create a well-rounded and effective workout plan that aligns with your goals. Patience, dedication, and a balanced approach to exercise and nutrition will contribute to steady and sustainable muscle growth over time.

How does fat leave the body?

When the body loses fat, it undergoes a process known as lipolysis, which involves the breakdown of triglycerides (the storage form of fat) into smaller molecules that can be used for energy. The byproducts of this process are then eliminated from the body through various mechanisms. Here's an overview of how fat leaves the body:

1. **Lipolysis:** Lipolysis is initiated when the body needs energy and doesn't have an immediate supply of calories from food. Hormones, such as adrenaline and noradrenaline, signal fat cells (adipocytes) to release stored triglycerides.

2. **Breakdown of Triglycerides:** Enzymes called lipases break down triglycerides into free fatty acids and glycerol. These smaller molecules are released into the bloodstream and transported to various tissues to be used as energy sources.

3. **Energy Production:** The free fatty acids and glycerol are taken up by cells, particularly muscle cells, where they undergo a process called beta-oxidation. This process occurs within the mitochondria of cells and generates energy in the form of adenosine triphosphate (ATP).

4. **Metabolism and Elimination:** The metabolic pathways in cells eventually convert the products of lipolysis into carbon dioxide (CO_2) and water (H_2O). The carbon dioxide is transported in the bloodstream and expelled from the body through the lungs when

you exhale. Water can be used by the body or eliminated through urine, sweat, and other bodily fluids.

5. **Breathing:** The majority of fat lost from the body is actually exhaled as carbon dioxide when you breathe. When fat molecules are broken down, the carbon atoms are released as carbon dioxide and exhaled as you breathe.

It's important to note that the process of fat loss occurs throughout the body and is not localized to specific areas. When the body loses weight, it draws energy from fat stores across various regions.

While the concept of fat being "burned" might conjure images of flames or smoke, it's actually a chemical process that results in the production of carbon dioxide and water. This process underscores the importance of a balanced diet, regular physical activity, and a healthy lifestyle for effective and sustainable fat loss.

What is the best way to maintain healthy skin as we age?

Maintaining healthy skin as you age requires a combination of proper skincare practices, a healthy lifestyle, and protecting your skin from external factors. Here are some key tips to help you maintain healthy skin as you get older:

1. **Protect Your Skin from the Sun:**

   - Apply sunscreen with at least SPF 30 daily, even on cloudy days.

   - Seek shade, especially during peak sun hours (10 a.m. to 4 p.m.).

   - Wear protective clothing, wide-brimmed hats, and sunglasses to shield your skin from UV rays.

2. **Stay Hydrated:**

   - Drink plenty of water throughout the day to keep your skin hydrated from within.

3. **Follow a Gentle Skincare Routine:**

   - Use a mild cleanser to cleanse your face morning and night.

   - Apply a moisturizer suitable for your skin type to keep your skin hydrated.

   - Use products with active ingredients like retinoids, hyaluronic acid, and antioxidants to address specific concerns.

4. **Avoid Harsh Products:**

   - Avoid products with harsh chemicals, fragrances, or alcohol that can strip your skin of its natural moisture.

5. **Eat a Nutrient-Rich Diet:**

   - Consume a diet rich in antioxidants, vitamins, and minerals. Foods like fruits, vegetables, whole grains, lean proteins, and healthy fats contribute to skin health.

6. **Stay Active:**

   - Regular physical activity promotes healthy circulation, which can contribute to a vibrant complexion.

7. **Get Adequate Sleep:**

   - Aim for 7-9 hours of quality sleep each night. Sleep is essential for skin repair and regeneration.

8. **Manage Stress:**

   - Chronic stress can affect your skin's health. Practice stress-reduction techniques like meditation, yoga, and deep breathing.

9. **Quit Smoking:**

   - Smoking accelerates skin aging by damaging collagen and elastin fibers. Quitting smoking can improve skin health.

10. **Limit Alcohol Consumption:**

- Excessive alcohol consumption can dehydrate your skin and lead to premature aging.

11. **Moisturize Regularly:**

- Use a moisturizer to keep your skin hydrated and prevent dryness, which can contribute to wrinkles.

12. **Regularly Exfoliate:**

- Gently exfoliate your skin to remove dead skin cells and promote cell turnover. However, avoid over-exfoliation, which can damage your skin.

13. **Hydrate Your Skin:**

- Use a hydrating serum or moisturizer with hyaluronic acid to maintain your skin's moisture balance.

14. **Protect Your Skin from Pollution:**

- In urban environments, consider using products that offer protection against environmental pollutants.

15. **Consult a Dermatologist:**

- Regular visits to a dermatologist can help you address specific skin concerns and receive personalized advice.

Remember that everyone's skin is unique, and what works best for one person may not work the same way for another. It's important to develop a skincare routine that suits your individual skin type and concerns. By combining healthy lifestyle habits with proper skincare practices, you can promote healthy and vibrant skin as you age.

How Do To Lose Fat

Losing fat involves a combination of regular exercise and a balanced, calorie-controlled diet. While I can't provide a complete program because while at Planet Fitness I cannot provide you with nutritional advice, I can give you a general outline for creating a fat loss program. Keep in mind that it's recommended to consult a healthcare professional before starting any new fitness or nutrition plan.

Here's a simple outline for a fat loss program:

1. **Set Clear Goals:** Define your fat loss goals in terms of pounds to lose, target body composition, and a reasonable timeframe.

2. **Calculate Daily Caloric Intake:** Determine your Basal Metabolic Rate (BMR) and Total Daily Energy Expenditure (TDEE) to find out how many calories you need to maintain your current weight. To lose fat, aim for a caloric deficit by consuming fewer calories than your TDEE.

3. **Design a Balanced Diet:** Create a diet plan that includes lean proteins, complex carbohydrates, healthy fats, and a variety of fruits and vegetables. Monitor portion sizes and consider using a food tracking app to help you stay on track.

4. **Monitor Macros:** Pay attention to macronutrient distribution. A common starting point is to aim for a split of around 40% carbohydrates, 30% protein, and 30% fat. Adjust these ratios based on your preferences and body's response.

5. **Stay Hydrated:** Drink plenty of water throughout the day to support metabolism and reduce feelings of hunger.

6. **Include Regular Exercise:** Incorporate a mix of cardiovascular exercise (e.g., walking, jogging, cycling) and strength training (e.g., weight lifting, bodyweight exercises). Aim for at least 150 minutes of moderate-intensity cardio per week and 2-3 days of strength training.

7. **High-Intensity Interval Training (HIIT):** Incorporate HIIT sessions to increase calorie burn and improve cardiovascular fitness. HIIT involves short bursts of intense exercise followed by periods of rest.

8. **Get Enough Sleep:** Prioritize sleep, aiming for 7-9 hours per night. Sleep is crucial for fat loss, recovery, and overall well-being.

9. **Monitor Progress:** Regularly track your weight, body measurements, and how your clothes fit. Remember that the scale isn't the only indicator of progress.

10. **Stay Consistent:** Consistency is key to long-term fat loss success. Make gradual, sustainable changes to your lifestyle.

11. **Seek Professional Guidance:** Consider working with a registered dietitian, nutritionist, or personal trainer who can tailor a program to your individual needs and provide expert guidance.

12. **Stay Patient and Positive:** Fat loss takes time and effort. Stay positive and patient, celebrating both small and significant milestones along the way.

Remember, losing fat is a gradual process, and everyone's journey is unique. Adapt the program to your preferences and listen to your body.

TDEE stands for Total Daily Energy Expenditure. It represents the total number of calories your body burns in a day, taking into account your basal metabolic rate (BMR) and the energy expended through physical activity. TDEE includes the calories you need to maintain your current weight, considering your activity level.

Here's a breakdown of the components that make up TDEE:

1. **Basal Metabolic Rate (BMR):** BMR is the number of calories your body needs to maintain basic physiological functions while at rest, such as breathing, circulating blood, and regulating body temperature. It's the energy required to keep your body functioning even if you're just lying in bed all day.

2. **Physical Activity Level (PAL):** PAL takes into account your daily activity level, including both

exercise and non-exercise activities (like walking, standing, and fidgeting). Different activity levels are usually categorized as sedentary, lightly active, moderately active, very active, or extremely active.

To calculate your TDEE, you generally use the Harris-Benedict equation or the Mifflin-St Jeor equation, both of which take into account your BMR and activity level:

Harris-Benedict Equation (for men): TDEE = BMR x Activity Multiplier

Harris-Benedict Equation (for women): TDEE = BMR x Activity Multiplier

Mifflin-St Jeor Equation (for men): TDEE = (10 * weight in kg) + (6.25 * height in cm) - (5 * age in years) + 5 x Activity Multiplier

Mifflin-St Jeor Equation (for women): TDEE = (10 * weight in kg) + (6.25 * height in cm) - (5 * age in years) - 161 x Activity Multiplier

The activity multiplier is usually determined based on your activity level:

- Sedentary (little or no exercise): BMR x 1.2

- Lightly active (light exercise/sports 1-3 days/week): BMR x 1.375

- Moderately active (moderate exercise/sports 3-5 days/week): BMR x 1.55

- Very active (hard exercise/sports 6-7 days a week): BMR x 1.725

- Extremely active (very hard exercise/sports, physical job, or training twice a day): BMR x 1.9

Once you calculate your TDEE, you can adjust your calorie intake to create a caloric deficit (if your goal is fat loss) or a surplus (if your goal is muscle gain). It's important to note that TDEE calculations are estimations, and individual variations can occur. Monitoring your progress and adjusting your approach as needed is crucial for achieving your goals.

Harris-Benedict Equation for Men (using pounds and inches): BMR = 66 + (6.2 * weight in pounds) + (12.7 * height in inches) - (6.76 * age in years)

Harris-Benedict Equation for Women (using pounds and inches): BMR = 655.1 + (4.35 * weight in pounds) + (4.7 * height in inches) - (4.7 * age in years)

After calculating your BMR using the appropriate formula above, you can then multiply.

Is a teaspoon of olive oil good for your health?

Yes, incorporating a teaspoon of olive oil into your diet can offer health benefits. Olive oil is known for its monounsaturated fatty acids, antioxidants, and other bioactive compounds that are linked to various positive effects on health. Here are some of the potential benefits of consuming olive oil:

1. **Heart Health:** Olive oil is rich in monounsaturated fats, which can help improve your heart health by reducing bad cholesterol levels (LDL cholesterol) and promoting good cholesterol (HDL cholesterol). It also contains antioxidants that have been associated with cardiovascular benefits.

2. **Anti-Inflammatory Properties:** Olive oil contains compounds such as polyphenols that have anti-inflammatory effects. Chronic inflammation is linked to various chronic diseases, so consuming olive oil may help mitigate inflammation.

3. **Antioxidant Benefits:** Olive oil is a source of antioxidants, such as vitamin E and polyphenols, which can help protect cells from oxidative stress and damage caused by free radicals.

4. **Weight Management:** Despite being calorie-dense, using moderate amounts of olive oil as a part of a balanced diet may help with weight management due to its potential to promote satiety and support metabolic health.

5. **Digestive Health:** Olive oil consumption has been associated with promoting healthy digestion and reducing the risk of gastrointestinal disorders.

6. **Brain Health:** The monounsaturated fats and antioxidants in olive oil may contribute to brain health and cognitive function.

7. **Skin Health:** The antioxidants and healthy fats in olive oil can potentially contribute to skin health by protecting against oxidative damage and supporting skin hydration.

It's important to note that while olive oil is a healthy fat source, it's still calorie-dense, so portion control is key. A teaspoon of olive oil contains around 40-50 calories, so incorporating it into your meals mindfully can help you enjoy its benefits without excessive calorie intake. Choose extra virgin olive oil for maximum health benefits, as it is less processed and retains more of its natural compounds.

Remember that a balanced and varied diet, along with other healthy lifestyle practices, contributes to overall well-being. Consult with a healthcare professional or a registered dietitian for personalized dietary recommendations based on your individual health needs and goals.

What fruits and vegetables have the highest antioxidant values?

Many fruits and vegetables are rich in antioxidants, which help protect cells from oxidative stress and support overall health. Here are some examples of fruits and vegetables that are known for their high antioxidant content:

Berries:

- Blueberries
- Strawberries
- Raspberries
- Blackberries
- Cranberries
- Goji berries
- Acai berries

Other Fruits:

- Pomegranates
- Cherries
- Apples (with the skin)
- Oranges and citrus fruits (e.g., oranges, grapefruits, lemons)
- Kiwi
- Grapes (especially red grapes)

Leafy Greens:

- Spinach
- Kale
- Swiss chard

- Collard greens

Other Vegetables:

- Bell peppers (especially red, orange, and yellow varieties)
- Broccoli
- Tomatoes
- Carrots
- Sweet potatoes

Legumes and Beans:

- Black beans
- Red kidney beans
- Pinto beans
- Lentils

Nuts and Seeds:

- Walnuts
- Pecans
- Almonds
- Flaxseeds
- Chia seeds

Spices:

- Cloves
- Cinnamon
- Turmeric

These foods are not only rich in antioxidants but also provide other essential nutrients such as vitamins, minerals, and dietary fiber. Keep in mind that different antioxidants offer various health benefits, so consuming a wide variety of colorful fruits and vegetables is recommended to ensure you're getting a diverse range of antioxidants.

Remember that it's the overall pattern of your diet that matters most for health. Incorporating a mix of these antioxidant-rich foods into your daily meals can contribute to better overall well-being.

What is a good age to get a shingles vaccination?

The shingles (herpes zoster) vaccine is recommended for adults aged 50 years and older to help prevent shingles and its complications. The vaccine is specifically designed to reduce the risk of developing shingles, as well as the severity and duration of symptoms if a person does get shingles.

There are two main types of shingles vaccines:

1. **Zoster Vaccine Live (Zostavax):** This vaccine was previously available but has been largely replaced by a newer, more effective vaccine.

2. **Shingrix:** Shingrix is the preferred shingles vaccine and is recommended by health authorities. It is a non-live vaccine and has shown to be highly effective at preventing shingles and its complications.

For Shingrix:

- The Centers for Disease Control and Prevention (CDC) recommends that adults aged 50 and older receive the Shingrix vaccine.
- The vaccine is administered in two doses, with the second dose given 2 to 6 months after the first dose.
- If you've previously had Zostavax, you should still receive the Shingrix vaccine, as it is more effective.

It's important to note that even if you've had shingles before, you can still benefit from the shingles vaccine to reduce the risk of a recurrence.

As always, it's a good idea to consult with your healthcare provider before getting any vaccine, especially if you have specific health conditions or concerns. Your healthcare provider can help determine the best timing for vaccination based on your individual health status and medical history.

What is a good age to get a pneumonia vaccination?

The pneumonia vaccine is recommended for adults at different ages based on their health conditions and risk factors. There are two main types of pneumonia vaccines: the pneumococcal conjugate vaccine (PCV13) and the pneumococcal polysaccharide vaccine (PPSV23). Here are the general recommendations for each vaccine:

1. **Pneumococcal Conjugate Vaccine (PCV13):**

    - The PCV13 vaccine is recommended for all adults aged 65 and older.

    - It is also recommended for adults aged 19 through 64 who have certain medical conditions that put them at higher risk for pneumonia, such as chronic lung disease, heart disease, diabetes, or a weakened immune system.

    - Some adults who have not previously received PCV13 and who are at high risk for pneumococcal disease due to certain medical conditions may need a dose of PCV13 before receiving PPSV23.

2. **Pneumococcal Polysaccharide Vaccine (PPSV23):**

    - The PPSV23 vaccine is recommended for all adults aged 65 and older.

    - It is also recommended for adults aged 19 through 64 who have certain medical conditions that increase their risk for pneumonia.

    - Adults aged 19 through 64 who smoke cigarettes should also receive PPSV23.

Additionally, if you are an adult aged 19 through 64 and you have a weakened immune system, are a smoker, or have other risk factors, your healthcare provider may recommend a combination of PCV13 and PPSV23 vaccines based on your individual situation.

It's important to note that these recommendations can vary based on specific health conditions, risk factors, and changes in guidelines over time. Therefore, it's best to consult with your healthcare provider to determine the appropriate timing and type of pneumonia vaccine for your situation. They can provide personalized recommendations based on your medical history and individual health needs.

Should I continue to get a COVID-19 Booster Shot?

As of my last knowledge update in September 2021, recommendations for COVID-19 booster shots have been evolving and can vary based on factors such as age, vaccination history, risk factors, and the emergence of new variants. It's important to refer to the most current guidance from reputable health authorities such as the Centers for Disease Control and Prevention (CDC), the World Health Organization (WHO), and your local public health department for the latest information.

As of my last update:

1. **Third Dose (Booster) for Certain Populations:** In some countries, third doses (boosters) of COVID-19 vaccines have been recommended for certain groups of individuals, such as those with weakened immune systems and those who are at higher risk of severe disease due to age or underlying health conditions.

2. **Emerging Variants:** The need for booster shots may be influenced by the emergence of new variants of the virus. Some variants may lead to reduced vaccine effectiveness over time, particularly against mild or moderate infections. Booster doses could help enhance protection, especially against variants.

3. **Mixing and Matching Vaccines:** Some places have explored the option of mixing and matching vaccines (using a different vaccine for the booster shot than the initial doses) to potentially enhance immunity.

4. **Global Equity:** While booster shots are being discussed in some countries, there's also a focus on ensuring equitable access to vaccines around the world, especially in regions where vaccination rates are still low.

Keep in mind that the situation is evolving, and recommendations may change based on new data and developments. If you're wondering about whether to get a COVID-19 booster shot, I recommend consulting your healthcare provider and referring to official health agencies for the latest guidance that's relevant to your location and circumstances. It's also important to follow any guidelines provided by your local public health authorities.

How important is sleep in maintaining overall fitness?

Sleep is a crucial component of maintaining overall fitness and well-being. It plays a significant role in various aspects of physical, mental, and emotional health. Here's why sleep is important for maintaining fitness:

1. **Physical Recovery:** During sleep, the body undergoes important repair and recovery processes. Muscles, tissues, and cells are repaired, and the body releases growth hormone, which is essential for muscle growth and repair.

2. **Muscle Growth:** Sleep is when the body repairs and builds new muscle tissue. Adequate sleep supports the growth and maintenance of lean muscle mass, which is important for overall fitness and metabolism.

3. **Energy Levels:** Quality sleep helps replenish energy stores and improves overall energy levels during waking hours. This is crucial for effective workouts and daily physical activities.

4. **Hormone Regulation:** Sleep is involved in regulating hormones related to appetite and metabolism. Poor sleep can disrupt hormone balance and potentially lead to weight gain or difficulty managing weight.

5. **Cognitive Function:** Sleep is essential for cognitive function, including memory, attention, concentration, and problem-solving abilities. These cognitive skills are important for effective workout planning and execution.

6. **Exercise Performance:** Getting enough restorative sleep can enhance exercise performance by improving coordination, reaction time, and overall mental and physical readiness.

7. **Injury Prevention:** Adequate sleep supports the body's ability to respond to stress and recover from workouts. Insufficient sleep increases the risk of injuries due to reduced physical and mental alertness.

8. **Immune Function:** Sleep is vital for a healthy immune system. Consistent sleep helps the body defend against infections and supports recovery from illnesses or injuries.

9. **Mood and Motivation:** Sleep has a direct impact on mood, emotional resilience, and motivation. Good mental health is essential for staying consistent with fitness goals.

10. **Recovery from Intense Workouts:** Intense workouts can cause micro-tears in muscles. Quality sleep is critical for the body's recovery process after such workouts.

11. **Overall Well-Being:** Regular, restorative sleep contributes to improved overall well-being, which

positively influences your ability to engage in physical activity and maintain fitness routines.

For optimal fitness and health benefits, aim for 7-9 hours of quality sleep each night. Establishing a consistent sleep schedule, creating a calming bedtime routine, and creating a sleep-conducive environment can help improve sleep quality. Prioritizing sleep alongside other elements of a healthy lifestyle, such as regular exercise and balanced nutrition, will contribute to your overall fitness journey.

Does exercise help with menopause symptoms?

Yes, exercise can be beneficial in managing and alleviating some of the symptoms associated with menopause. Menopause is a natural phase of life that occurs as a woman's reproductive hormones decline, typically around the age of 45 to 55. During this transition, women may experience a range of physical and emotional changes, including hot flashes, mood swings, weight gain, reduced bone density, and decreased muscle mass.

Regular exercise can have several positive effects on menopause symptoms:

1. **Hot Flashes:** Some studies suggest that regular physical activity can help reduce the frequency and severity of hot flashes. Exercise may improve the body's temperature regulation and hormonal balance.

2. **Mood Improvement:** Exercise has been shown to have positive effects on mood and emotional well-being. It can help reduce feelings of anxiety, depression, and irritability that may be heightened during menopause.

3. **Weight Management:** Menopause can be associated with weight gain and changes in body composition. Engaging in regular physical activity, including both cardiovascular exercise and strength training, can help manage weight and preserve lean muscle mass.

4. **Bone Health:** Menopause is associated with a decline in bone density, which increases the risk of osteoporosis. Weight-bearing exercises like walking, jogging, and resistance training can help maintain bone density and reduce the risk of fractures.

5. **Cardiovascular Health:** Cardiovascular risks, including an increased risk of heart disease, can become more significant during and after menopause. Exercise improves cardiovascular fitness, lowers blood pressure, and helps maintain healthy cholesterol levels.

6. **Energy Levels:** Regular exercise can boost energy levels and combat feelings of fatigue that may be associated with menopause.

7. **Sleep Quality:** Menopause can disrupt sleep patterns. Engaging in physical activity can promote better sleep by improving sleep quality and reducing insomnia.

8. **Brain Health:** Exercise is associated with cognitive benefits, including improved memory and cognitive function. These benefits can be particularly important during menopause when some women may experience cognitive changes.

When incorporating exercise into your routine during menopause, consider the following tips:

- Choose activities you enjoy to increase adherence.

- Include a mix of cardiovascular exercises (e.g., walking, swimming, cycling) and strength training.

- Aim for at least 150 minutes of moderate-intensity aerobic activity per week, along with muscle-strengthening exercises on two or more days.

- Listen to your body and choose activities that align with your fitness level and any health considerations.

- Stay hydrated and practice good nutrition to support your exercise routine and overall health.

Before starting a new exercise program, especially if you have underlying health conditions, it's a good idea to consult with a healthcare provider to ensure that your chosen activities are safe and appropriate for your individual situation.

What are the best exercises to maintain balance from falling as we age?

Maintaining balance is crucial as we age to prevent falls and injuries. Incorporating balance exercises into your routine can help improve stability and reduce the risk of falls. Here are some effective exercises to help maintain balance as you age:

1. **Standing on One Leg:**

    - Stand near a wall or sturdy surface for support if needed.
    - Lift one leg off the ground and balance on the other leg.
    - Hold for 15-30 seconds and then switch legs.
    - As you progress, try to increase the time you can balance on each leg.

2. **Heel-to-Toe Walk:**

    - Imagine walking on a tightrope.
    - Place one foot in front of the other so that the heel of the front foot touches the toes of the back foot.
    - Take a step forward in this manner, alternating feet.
    - Perform this exercise in a straight line and gradually increase the distance you walk.

3. **Tai Chi:**

   - Tai Chi is a low-impact, flowing martial art that emphasizes balance, coordination, and relaxation.
   - Practicing Tai Chi regularly can improve balance, flexibility, and overall body awareness.

4. **Yoga:**

   - Yoga poses that challenge your balance, such as Tree Pose and Warrior III, can help improve stability.
   - Yoga also focuses on flexibility and strength, which are important for overall balance.

5. **Single Leg Squats:**

   - Stand on one leg with the other leg lifted slightly in front of you.
   - Slowly lower yourself into a squat while keeping your lifted leg extended in front.
   - Press through the heel of your supporting foot to return to the starting position.
   - Repeat on the other leg.

6. **Leg Swings:**

   - Hold onto a sturdy support if needed.
   - Swing one leg forward and backward while maintaining your balance.

- Gradually increase the range of motion and the number of swings before switching legs.

7. **Seated Marching:**

   - Sit on a sturdy chair with your feet flat on the ground.
   - Lift one knee as high as comfortable, then lower it down.
   - Repeat on the other side, alternating legs like you're marching in place.

8. **Resistance Band Exercises:**

   - Using a resistance band for exercises like leg lifts and side leg raises can help strengthen the muscles that support your balance.

9. **Stability Ball Exercises:**

   - Exercises performed on a stability ball, such as seated marches or gentle pelvic tilts, can engage your core and improve balance.

10. **Water Workouts:**

   - Water aerobics or swimming can be great options for low-impact balance exercises that also provide resistance.

When performing balance exercises, make sure to have a stable surface nearby to hold onto if needed. Start with exercises that match your current fitness level and gradually progress as your balance improves. If you have any medical conditions or concerns, consult with a healthcare provider or a fitness professional before starting a new exercise routine.

Here is a total body workout using only your body weight.

Here's a total body workout that utilizes only bodyweight exercises. This workout targets different muscle groups and provides a well-rounded workout without the need for equipment. Remember to warm up before starting and cool down afterward.

Warm-Up: Perform 5-10 minutes of light cardio, such as jogging in place, jumping jacks, or dynamic stretches like arm circles and leg swings.

Workout: Perform each exercise for the designated number of repetitions or time, and then move on to the next exercise. Rest for 1-2 minutes between sets and exercises if needed.

1. **Push-Ups:**

   - Reps: 10-15

   - Target: Chest, shoulders, triceps, core

2. **Bodyweight Squats:**

   - Reps: 15-20

   - Target: Quadriceps, hamstrings, glutes

3. **Plank:**

   - Hold: 30-60 seconds

   - Target: Core, shoulders, back

4. **Lunges:**

   - Reps: 10-15 each leg

   - Target: Quadriceps, hamstrings, glutes

5. **Tricep Dips:**

   - Reps: 12-15

   - Target: Triceps, shoulders

6. **Bridge/Hip Thrusts:**

   - Reps: 15-20

   - Target: Glutes, hamstrings, lower back

7. **Mountain Climbers:**

   - Reps: 20-30 (each leg)

   - Target: Core, shoulders, legs

8. **Supermans:**

   - Reps: 12-15

   - Target: Lower back, glutes, upper back

9. **Side Planks:**

   - Hold: 20-30 seconds each side

   - Target: Core, obliques, shoulders

10. **Burpees:**

    - Reps: 8-10

- Target: Full-body conditioning

Cool-Down: Spend 5-10 minutes stretching your muscles, focusing on areas that were worked during the workout. Include static stretches for major muscle groups such as hamstrings, quadriceps, calves, chest, and shoulders.

Remember to perform each exercise with proper form and technique. If you're new to exercise or have any underlying health conditions, consider consulting a fitness professional or healthcare provider before starting a new workout routine. As you progress, you can adjust the number of repetitions or time to match your fitness level and goals.

Epilogue

In the journey of this book, we've explored the intricate dance between body and mind, the symphony of movement and nourishment, and the powerful transformations that unfold when we commit to our own well-being. From the first steps taken on the path of fitness to the milestones reached, the pursuit of health is a deeply personal odyssey, guided by determination and fueled by passion.

As you close these pages, remember that fitness is not a destination but a lifelong voyage—a journey of self-discovery, resilience, and growth. The story doesn't end here; it continues with every choice you make, every challenge you overcome, and every small victory that becomes a part of your narrative.

May this book serve as a compass, leading you through the ups and downs, the plateaus and breakthroughs, and the moments of doubt and triumph. Embrace the wisdom you've gained, and let it empower you to step confidently into your own journey, forging a path of health, vitality, and happiness.

With each sunrise, you have the opportunity to redefine your limits, reshape your habits, and sculpt the masterpiece that is your body and soul. May your story be one of strength, courage, and boundless possibility.

Here's to embracing the joy of movement, savoring the nourishment of wholesome choices, and embarking on a life rich with vitality. The final chapter is yours to write, and the journey, as it always has been, is yours to own.

Wishing you the strength to climb every mountain, the grace to navigate every curve, and the resilience to savor every step of the magnificent journey that is fitness."

Every Day Is A Holy Day/Holiday. Every Meal Is A Feast!

Yours Truly
Bruce H. Dobbs

For more information on fitness go to:
www.yourphenomenallife.net